ANAESTHESIA,
RECOVERY AND INTENSIVE CARE

MODERN NURSING SERIES

General Editors

A. J. HARDING RAINS M.S., F.R.C.S.
Professor of Surgery, Charing Cross Hospital Medical School, University of London; Honorary Consultant Surgeon, Charing Cross Hospital; Honorary Consultant Surgeon to the Army.

VALERIE HUNT S.R.N., S.C.M., O.N.D., R.N.T.
Formerly District Nursing Officer, Southmead Health District, Avon Area Health Authority (Teaching); Past Chairman General Nursing Council of England and Wales.

A SELECTION OF TITLES AVAILABLE AS PAPERBACKS

Ear, Nose and Throat Surgery and Nursing
R PRACY M.B., B.S., F.R.C.S.,
J SIEGLER M.B., B.S., D.L.O., F.R.C.S.
P M. STELL M.B., F.R.C.S.
J ROGERS M.A., F.R.C.S.

Neurology
EDWIN R. BICKERSTAFF M.D., M.R.C.P.

Obstetrics and Gynaecology
GORDON W. GARLAND M.D., F.R.C.O.G.
JOAN M. E. QUIXLEY S.R.N.

Principles of Medicine and Medical Nursing
J. C. HOUSTON M.D., F.R.C.P.
MARION STOCKDALE S.R.N.

Principles of Surgery and Surgical Nursing
SELWYN TAYLOR D.M., M.Ch., F.R.C.S.

Physiology for Nurses
DERYCK TAVERNER M.B.E., M.D., F.R.C.P.

Venereology and Genito-Urinary Medicine
R. D. CATTERALL F.R.C.P. (Edin.)

Psychology and Psychiatry for Nurses
PETER DALLY M.B., F.R.C.P., D.P.M.
HEATHER HARRINGTON S.R.N., R.M.N.

Emergency and Acute Care
A. J. HARDING RAINS M.S., F.R.C.S.
VALERIE HUNT S.R.N., S.C.M.
KEITH REYNOLDS F.R.C.S.

Microbiology in Patient Care
H. I. WINNER M.D., F.R.C.P., F.R.C.Path.

ANAESTHESIA,

RECOVERY AND INTENSIVE CARE

D. A. BUXTON HOPKIN, M.D.(Lond.), F.F.A.R.C.S.
Consultant Anaesthetist,
Charing Cross Hospital; Honorary Consultant Anaesthetist,
St. Thomas's Hospital;
formerly Lecturer in Anaesthesia,
University of Malaya, Singapore

HODDER AND STOUGHTON
London Sydney Auckland Toronto

ISBN 0 340 09898 8

First published 1970. Reprinted 1975 with revisions, 1976, 1978, 1981

Printed and bound in Great Britain for Hodder and Stoughton Educational, a division of Hodder and Stoughton, Ltd., London by T. and A. Constable Ltd., Edinburgh

TO MY WIFE

PREFACE

Anaesthesia has often been compared with air travel because 'take-off' and 'touchdown' have much in common with induction of anaesthesia and recovery, both being moments of maximal hazard calling for a high degree of technical knowledge and imposing a heavy responsibility on anaesthetists and pilots. This is indeed true, but the analogy can be taken a step further. Pilots and anaesthetists both depend on a number of other people before, during and afterwards, who make a significant contribution to the safety of passengers and patients and who by their personal efforts encourage confidence in what otherwise could be a traumatic and distressing experience.

The object of this book is to present the background knowledge of anaesthesia necessary for all those who assist anaesthetists or who come into personal contact with their patients, whether in the ward, the operating theatre or the recovery room. Certain sections may be helpful for nurses who are responsible for the preparation and after-care of patients undergoing anaesthesia. Other parts will interest those whose duties include assistance in the technical aspects of anaesthesia in the operating suite, whether nurses or theatre technicians.

The book could also provide pre-registration house officers and senior medical students with a brief introduction to the aims and objects of the practice of anaesthesia. Chapters on Intensive Care and the Treatment of Respiratory Failure have also been included because in some hospitals Recovery and Intensive Care run side by side and because anaesthetists are becoming increasingly involved in providing these services.

ACKNOWLEDGEMENTS

The author feels very indebted to several people who have assisted in the preparation of this book.

The Editor in Chief, Professor A. J. Harding Rains, has given constant encouragement and valuable practical advice during the preparation of the manuscript. The Anaesthetic Sisters at Fulham Hospital, Miss Hallinan and Miss A. Sneddon; the Chief Anaesthetic Technician at Lambeth Hospital, Mr F. Wheadon, F.I.O.T.; the Recovery Room Sisters at Lambert Hospital, Miss A. Brown and Miss M. Higgon; the former Sister in charge of the Intensive Care Unit at Charing Cross Hospital, Miss S. Morton, have all made helpful suggestions. The secretaries to the Anaesthetic Department at Charing Cross Hospital, Miss F. Westerman and her successor, Miss S. Curd, and Professor Rains' former secretary, Miss S. Ong, have shared the burden of typing and re-typing the manuscript several times.

The artist, Mr H. Grayshon Lumby, has brought the book to life with his splendid illustrations, so ably prepared from thumbnail sketches or illustrations from the catalogues of British Oxygen Co., Medical and Industrial Equipment Ltd, Oxygenaire and Airmed Ltd, to whom thanks are due for their permission to use their material in this way.

Finally, Mr Robert Coates and the production staff of The English Universities Press who have given valuable assistance and guidance in the proof stages, and set out the text with admirable order and clarity.

CONTENTS

PREFACE vii

1 GENERAL ANAESTHESIA
Some questions and answers 1

2 PREPARATION OF THE PATIENT—I 13
Physical examination and assessment 13
Drugs causing adverse reactions with anaesthetics 17
Pre-operative assessment for emergency surgery 18

3 PREPARATION OF THE PATIENT—II 20
Pre-anaesthetic medication and transfer to the Operating Suite 20
Preparation of children 22
Final preparations on the day of operation 24
Preparation of day patients 26

4 THE ANAESTHETIC ROOM—I 29
Control of access to the anaesthetic room 29
Contents of the anaesthetic room 29
Anaesthetic apparatus 30
Other types of anaesthetic apparatus 41

5 THE ANAESTHETIC ROOM—II 42
Breathing attachments 42
Carbon dioxide absorption apparatus 46
Suction equipment 51
Airways 53
Mouth gags 57

6 THE ANAESTHETIC ROOM—III 59
Equipment for endotracheal anaesthesia 59
Modified equipment for infants and small children 69

7 THE ANAESTHETIC ROOM—IV 74

Intravenous equipment 74
Fluids for intravenous therapy 81

8 THE ANAESTHETIC ROOM—V 85

Monitoring equipment 85
Prevention of fire and explosions 90

9 THE ANAESTHETIC ROOM—VI 92

Organisation and preparations for anaesthesia 92
Cleaning and sterilisation of equipment 96

10 POSITION OF THE PATIENT ON THE OPERATING TABLE 99

General rules 99
Common positions for surgery 99

11 THE RECOVERY ROOM—I 104

Planning and organisation 104
Nursing procedures 107

12 THE RECOVERY ROOM—II 113

Anaesthetic complications 113
Complications arising from the operation 115

13 RESPIRATORY FAILURE—I: THE PHYSIOLOGY OF NORMAL RESPIRATION 118

Ventilation 120
Diffusion 122
Perfusion 122

14 RESPIRATORY FAILURE—II: THE CAUSES AND THE PRINCIPLES OF TREATMENT 124

Types of respiratory failure 124
Principles of treatment 127
Oxygen therapy 127
Hyperbaric oxygen therapy 131

15 RESPIRATORY FAILURE—III: VENTILATORS 134

Advantages and disadvantages of volume-cycled and pressure-cycled machines 135

Treatment with a ventilator 135
Classification of ventilators 137

16 RESPIRATORY FAILURE—IV 138
Indications for tracheostomy 138
Advantages of tracheostomy 139
Instruments 139
Operative technique 141

17 RESPIRATORY FAILURE—V 142
Making contact with the patient 142
General care 142
Endotracheal suction 143
Chest physiotherapy 144

18 CARDIAC ARREST 146
Causes 146
Diagnosis 147
Principles of treatment 148
Organisation of treatment for acute cardiac arrest 153

19 INTENSIVE CARE UNIT 156
Advantages and disadvantages of an Intensive Care Unit 156
General arrangement 157
Type of patient 157
Problems of organisation and administration 158
Nursing care 158
Some conditions met in Intensive Care Units 162

20 LOCAL ANAESTHESIA 166
Methods 166
Drugs 168
Equipment 170
Care of patients 173

21 ANALGESIA AND ANAESTHESIA DURING CHILDBIRTH 175

22 DRUGS AND THEIR USES 182

INDEX 192

1 GENERAL ANAESTHESIA

The speed with which an anaesthetist can bring about the sudden change from full consciousness and awareness to immobility and oblivion can, at first sight, be frightening and mysterious. In bygone days, such powers would have been condemned as witchcraft. Even today, the anaesthetist retains some of the aura of a sorcerer endowed with magical powers which can control the capacity of the individual 'to speak, move and have his being'. To anyone watching an anaesthetist at work for the first time, many questions must come to mind—what is he giving the patient? Why does he need that tube? How does he know when to stop injecting? When will the patient recover? This chapter will attempt to answer some of these questions.

WHAT IS 'GENERAL' ANAESTHESIA?

The word 'Anaesthesia' was invented by Oliver Wendell Holmes to describe the condition of a patient rendered temporarily unconscious and insensitive to the pain of surgical operations following inhalation of ether vapour or nitrous-oxide gas ('Laughing Gas'). Subsequently, the discovery of another method of securing freedom from the pain of surgery *without* loss of consciousness, by injecting drugs which paralysed the nerves around the operative field imposed the necessity of distinguishing the two methods. *General* anaesthesia became the term used to delineate the method involving loss of consciousness whilst *Local* anaesthesia described the method of securing freedom from pain confined to the operation area although the patient remained awake. Some authorities prefer the term *Local Analgesia* because they maintain that the use of the term *Anaesthesia* implies loss of consciousness.

Anaesthesia has become a special branch of medicine which embraces many responsibilities including pre-operative assessment of patients, supervision of recovery, and intensive care. Those who devote their time exclusively to anaesthesia are known as *Anaesthetists.*

In some countries where nurses and technicians are allowed to administer anaesthesia the speciality of anaesthesia has become known as *Anaesthesiology* and the anaesthetist as the *Anaesthesiologist*.

HOW DO ANAESTHETICS AFFECT BRAIN CELLS?

Anaesthetics interrupt the processes whereby brain cells obtain energy from oxygen and glucose for the generation of nerve impulses. The interruption of function is temporary, and reversible. The return of normal activity, known as *Reversible Action*, is a property common to all anaesthetics, which distinguishes them from poisons of the nervous system such as potassium cyanide whose interference with oxygen utilisation is total and permanent.

WHY DO GENERAL ANAESTHETICS DEPRESS THE BRAIN?

The brain is more susceptible than other parts of the body to anaesthetic agents for three reaons:
(1) The brain *receives* proportionately more blood than other parts of the body by virtue of its generous blood supply;
(2) The brain *absorbs* more anaesthetic than other parts because fatty 'Lipoids' constitute the 75% of the 'White matter' (Myelin) of the brain, and all anaesthetic agents have a high affinity for fatty substances;
(3) The nerve cells responsible for the conscious state are the smallest and most delicate in the body and are hence the first to be affected by anaesthetics. The larger cells are depressed relatively late in anaesthesia. For example, those responsible for respiration continue functioning until the point of overdose is approached.

HOW IS GENERAL ANAESTHESIA PRODUCED?

Anaesthetics can be introduced into the body in three ways: through a *vein*, through the *lungs*, or by the *rectum*. Whichever route is used, the drug eventually reaches the circulation which carries it to the brain.

Intravenous anaesthesia is the commonest way of inducing unconsciousness. It is effective within 30 seconds and is not an unpleasant experience. In the aged or very ill patients, some respiratory and circulatory depression may follow intravenous induction and on these occasions anaesthesia by inhalation may be preferred.

Inhalation anaesthesia is induced by inhalation of the vapour of a liquid anaesthetic or of an anaesthetic gas. Although safe and reliable, it is unpleasant for the patient who resents a mask put over the face. Ether has an irritant odour and when inhaled may evoke feelings of suffocation.

Rectal anaesthesia. The rectal route is used to induce unconsciousness in apprehensive children, for it can be carried out in bed in the ward. *Ether*, dissolved in olive oil has been used for this purpose. *Tribromethanol* ('Avertin') was a popular agent but has been displaced by *Thiopentone* which is now available in a pack prepared for rectal use.

WHAT ARE THE COMMON INTRAVENOUS ANAESTHETICS?

The common intravenous agents are the barbiturate derivatives *thiopentone* (Intraval) and *methohexitone* (Brietal), prepared in powder form for solution in sterile water before use; and non-barbiturates *propanimid* (Epontol) and CT 1341 (Althesin) a steroid preparation. Brietal, Epontol, and Althesin have a short action suitable for casualty departments. The use of Ketalar is limited in Great Britain to small children who are said not to be affected by dreaming and psychic disturbances during recovery.

WHAT ARE THE COMMON INHALATION AGENTS?

Inhalational agents are either (1) *gaseous* at room temperature or (2) *liquids* with a boiling point well below that of water giving off vapour when oxygen or air is bubbled through them at room temperature.

WHAT ARE THE GASEOUS ANAESTHETICS?

The common gaseous anaesthetics are *cyclopropane* and *nitrous oxide* which are stored in cylinders under pressure in a liquid form. Cyclopropane, being very potent and only used in small amounts, comes in small *orange cylinders*. Nitrous oxide, a weak agent of which large quantities are used, is stored in *large blue cylinders*.

Cyclopropane is inflammable, and explosive when mixed with oxygen, hence it must not be used in the presence of diathermy or a cautery.

WHAT ARE THE LIQUID ANAESTHETICS?

Ether, trichlorethylene ('Trilene') and halothane ('Fluothane') are the common liquid anaesthetics. All have a boiling point below that of water and give off a vapour at room temperature, each detectable by a characteristic smell. Passage of air or oxygen through the liquid enclosed in a glass jar or metal container, known as a *vaporiser*, is used to increase the rate of vaporisation (page 30).

Ether has an unpleasant choking odour, but it has a high margin of safety even in unskilled hands. Prolonged etherisation causes post-operative depression and vomiting. Like cyclopropane, ether is inflammable, and explosive when mixed with oxygen (page 90).

Trichlorethylene ('Trilene') is coloured blue to distinguish it from commercial preparations widely used in the dry cleaning industry. It has a non-irritating and sweetish smell. Anaesthesia is not usually induced with trichlorethylene because of its slow rate of vaporisation, and it is more often employed to supplement the weak anaesthetic properties of nitrous oxide by its predominant analgesic action, after induction of anaesthesia with an intravenous agent such as thiopentone. The inhalation of small quantities (0·5% in air) although not accompanied by loss of consciousness, is sufficient to relieve pain, and is used for this purpose during childbirth (page 176).

Halothane ('Fluothane') was introduced into anaesthesia in 1955 after extensive research by British chemists for a volatile anaesthetic agent that was neither explosive nor inflammable. In the relatively few years since its introduction halothane has become very popular and together with nitrous oxide is more often employed to maintain anaesthesia than any other agent. The reasons for its popularity are lack of irritation of the respiratory tract making for smooth anaesthesia; effectiveness in low concentration; rapid recovery after administration, with absence of unwelcome side effects such as nausea, vomiting or circulatory or respiratory depression. Allegations that it can cause liver damage remain unproven, but it has been suggested that repeated administration increases the chance of jaundice. As however operative mortality is lower with halothane than any other agent, it will undoubtedly retain its popularity.

Methoxyfluorane ('Penthrane'). Methoxyfluorane is similar to halothane but vaporises less readily, so that induction and recovery are slower. Like trichlorethylene it has analgesic properties in low concentration. Methoxyfluorane has a sweet smell which closely resembles that of a brand of chewing gum known as 'Juicy Fruit'.

WHAT IS MAINTENANCE OF ANAESTHESIA?

The course of anaesthesia following induction is known as the 'maintenance' period.

WHAT AGENTS ARE USED TO MAINTAIN ANAESTHESIA?

Maintenance of anaesthesia after intravenous induction is by means of inhalational agents: nitrous oxide and oxygen from an anaesthetic machine with additions of small amounts of halothane, trichlorethylene, or ether; or by intermittent intravenous injection of addictive analgesics like pethidine. Muscle relaxants are added to produce muscle relaxation for abdominal surgery. Inhalational agents allow more precise control than intravenous anaesthetics, being eliminated by a physical process from the lungs whilst breakdown of intravenous anaesthetics depends on slower metabolic processes which are depressed in toxic states or as the result of operative shock.

WHAT IS A MUSCLE RELAXANT?

A muscle relaxant paralyses and relaxes voluntary muscles, but has no adverse effect on the brain or circulation.

A muscle relaxant is necessary to prevent contraction of the abdominal muscles during abdominal surgery so that the surgeon can examine or operate on its contents. Formerly the production of abdominal muscular relaxation required large doses of inhalational anaesthetics like ether which, within a short time, depressed the circulation and caused considerable post-operative morbidity. Muscle relaxants have made such large doses unnecessary, and reduced the hazards of abdominal surgery. Short acting muscle relaxants are commonly employed to relax the vocal cords prior to passage of an endotracheal tube.

HOW DOES A MUSCLE RELAXANT PARALYSE MUSCLES?

Muscle relaxants cause paralysis by interfering with neuromuscular transmission, i.e. the process whereby a nerve impulse produces muscle contraction.

HOW DOES NEUROMUSCULAR TRANSMISSION TAKE PLACE?

The motor nerve fibre divides into several small branches which end on the surface of the muscle fibres as structures called 'motor end plates'. Nerve impulses liberate acetyl choline at the motor end plate,

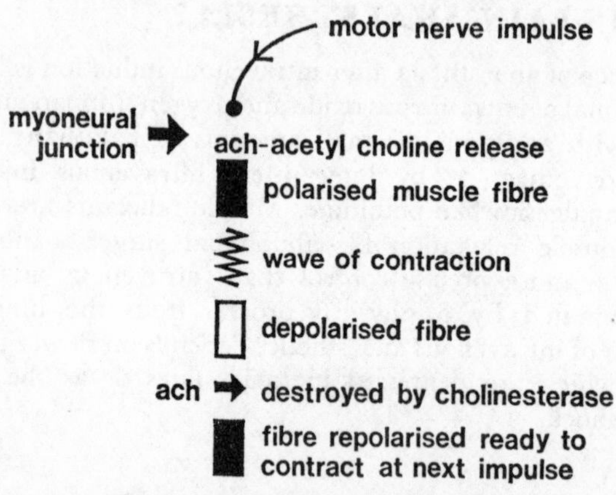

Fig. 1 Normal muscle contraction

which induces an electrical disturbance ('action potential'). During the passage of the potential and the subsequent contraction the muscle fibre is said to be '*polarised*'. *After* contraction it becomes '*depolarised*' and unresponsive to further stimuli until an enzyme 'Cholinesterase' has destroyed acetyl choline (Fig. 1).

HOW DO MUSCLE RELAXANTS PREVENT NEUROMUSCULAR TRANSMISSION?

Muscle relaxants interfere with neuromuscular transmission in one of two ways:

(1) *By preventing access of acetyl choline to the muscle fibre.* Molecules of the relaxant 'compete' with acetyl choline for receptors at the motor

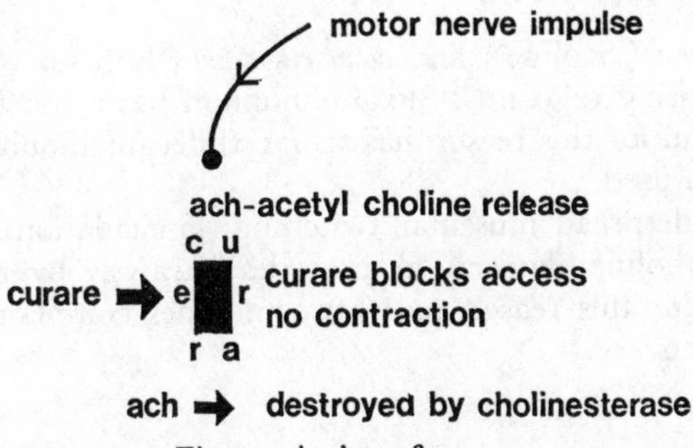

Fig. 2 Action of curare

end plates (Fig. 2), thus preventing contraction. This is called *competitive blockade.*

(2) *By intensifying the action of acetyl choline.* The muscle contracts normally, but remains relaxed and unresponsive to stimuli ('depolarised') because the muscle relaxant unlike acetyl choline is *not*

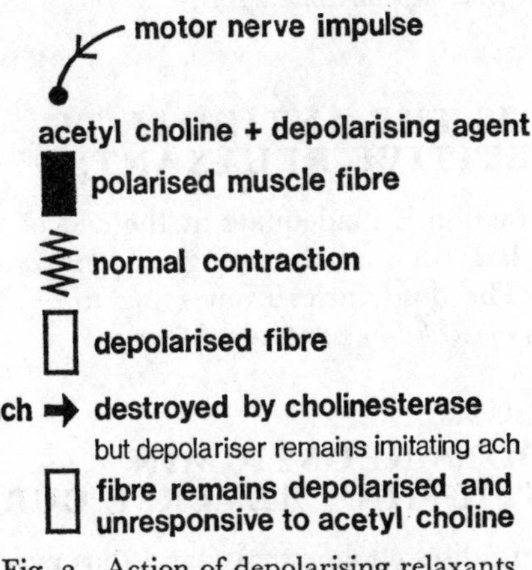

Fig. 3 Action of depolarising relaxants

destroyed by cholinesterase, and keeps the fibre depolarised (Fig. 3). Such relaxants are known as *depolarising relaxants.*

WHICH MUSCLE RELAXANTS ACT BY COMPETITIVE BLOCKADE?

Curare ('Tubarine'); *gallamine* ('Flaxedil'); *pancuronium bromide* ('Pavulon'), and *toxiferine* ('Alloferin') are *competitive blockers.*

WHICH ARE DEPOLARISING RELAXANTS?

Suxamethonium ('Scoline') and *decamethonium* ('Eulissin', 'Syncurine') are depolarising relaxants. Suxamethonium has a shorter duration of action and for this reason has replaced decamethonium which is now seldom used.

Note: Widespread muscular twitching (fasciculation)—(evidence of acetyl choline-like action) precedes paralysis by depolarising relaxants. For this reason patients sometimes complain of muscle pains on recovery.

ARE THERE ANTIDOTES TO MUSCLE RELAXANTS?

Full recovery may be expected from the effects of muscle relaxants, the time varying from 30–40 minutes for curare to 5–10 minutes for Scoline.

Antidotes are available to hasten recovery from *competitive* relaxants, but *not from depolarising agents.*

WHAT IS THE ANTIDOTE TO COMPETITIVE RELAXANTS?

If muscle contraction is inadequate at the end of an operation for which curare has been used neostigmin ('Prostigmin') is given intravenously. The dose varies from 1 mg to 2·5 mg given intravenously, *always preceded by atropine* 0·6–1 *mg.*

HOW DOES NEOSTIGMIN ('PROSTIGMIN') REVERSE CURARE?

Neostigmin neutralises cholinesterase and thus prevents destruction of acetyl choline which consequently accumulates in sufficient quantity to displace curare from the myoneural junction allowing resumption of normal muscle contraction (Fig. 4).

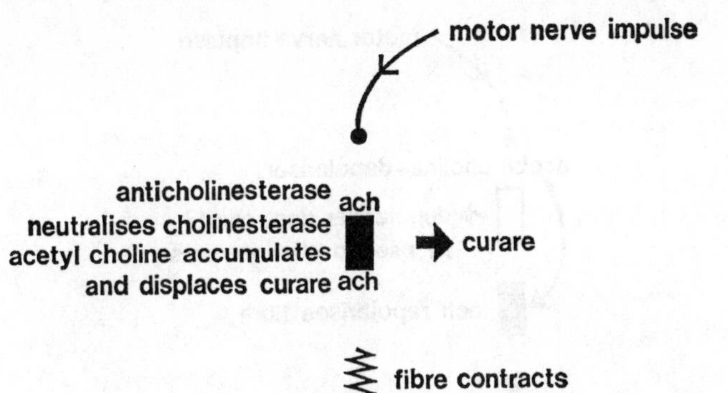

Fig. 4 Reversal of curare by anticholinesterase

WHY IS IT NECESSARY TO GIVE ATROPINE WITH NEOSTIGMIN ('PROSTIGMIN')?

Atropine should always be administered before neostigmin ('Prostigmin') to neutralise the effect of the excess of acetylcholine on the heart rate, which it slows and may cause cardiac arrest. Atropine increases the heart rate by reducing the activity of the vagus nerve thus avoiding this complication. Following administration of atropine and neostigmin ('Prostigmin'); the pulse should be observed with care. If the rate falls below 50 per minute, more atropine is needed.

IS THERE AN ANTIDOTE TO A DEPOLARISING RELAXANT?

There is no antidote to depolarising relaxants which are destroyed in the blood stream by an enzyme known as *pseudocholinesterase* (Fig. 5). Some patients (about 1 in 3,000) lack this enzyme. After administration of suxamethonium, delay in recovery occurs because it is not destroyed until normal disintegration occurs. The time taken will depend on the total dose administered and paralysis may persist for several hours. The condition is not dangerous provided that efficient artificial respiration (preferably with a ventilator) is carried out until full recovery of muscle contraction takes place.

Recovery can be accelerated by transfusion of compatible fresh blood containing *pseudo-cholinesterase*. Fresh blood is essential because pseudo-cholinesterase becomes inactive in stored blood. As the condition (lack of pseudo-cholinesterase) is hereditary, it is unwise to accept a relative of the patient as a donor.

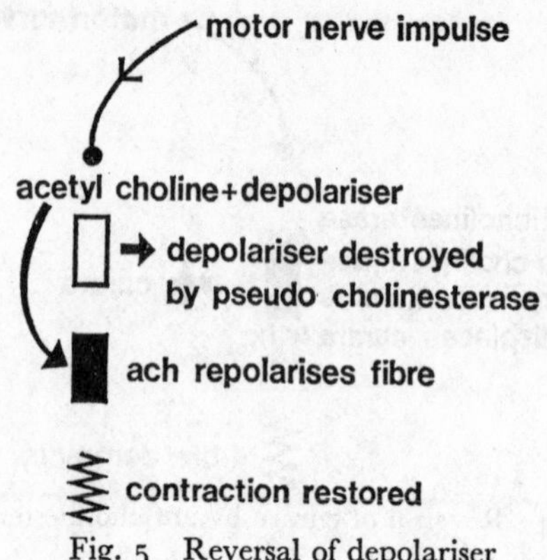

Fig. 5 Reversal of depolariser

WHAT IS ENDOTRACHEAL ANAESTHESIA?

Endotracheal anaesthesia is a method of maintaining anaesthesia by means of a curved rubber tube (endotracheal tube) introduced into the trachea and connected to the gas supply of the anaesthetic apparatus (page 30).

WHY IS AN ENDOTRACHEAL TUBE NECESSARY?

The original purpose of an endotracheal tube was to prevent blood passing into the trachea and lungs during operations on the nose, mouth and throat. The method was developed by Sir Ivan Magill and Dr Stanley Rowbotham to facilitate plastic surgery of the nose and face on severely maimed soldiers during the latter part of the First World War—for this reason endotracheal tubes are known as Magill's tubes.

Endotracheal intubation became a routine procedure after the introduction of muscle relaxants, not only to prevent inhalation of regurgitated gastric contents but to allow inflation of the lungs since subjects paralysed by a relaxant (*a*) cannot breathe and (*b*) cannot close the larynx by contracting the vocal cords.

SUMMARY

Modern anaesthesia consists of:

(1) *Induction of unconsciousness* with a small amount of intravenous anaesthetic.

(2) *Maintenance of unconsciousness* with inhalational agents: nitrous

oxide with added trilene, halothane, ether or intravenous opiate analgesics.

Reflex movement and *muscle rigidity* are prevented: (i) by increase in concentration of anaesthetic (halothane, trilene); (ii) by intravenous addictive analgesics (opiates) and (iii) by muscle relaxants.

Endotracheal tubes: (i) protect the lungs against aspiration through paralysed vocal cords, and (ii) allow inflation of the lungs following paralysis by relaxants.

HOW UNCONSCIOUS IS THE PATIENT?

Reflex movements following cutting the skin do not necessarily indicate consciousness or ability to feel pain.

The part of the brain responsible for consciousness is situated at the upper end of the brain stem just before it divides to support the cerebral hemispheres. The brain cells in this area are susceptible to the depressant effects of small concentrations of anaesthetics but the larger cells of the sensory and motor cortex of the cerebral hemispheres are more resistant. Under light anaesthesia cells receiving pain impulses continue to respond to pain stimuli and cause a discharge from the cells in the motor cortex to the motor pathways to the muscles which, on reaching a certain degree of intensity, causes involuntary movement although consciousness is no longer present.

Anaesthetists used to estimate the depth of anaesthesia by observing changes in respiratory rhythm and the sequence of the disappearance of reflex activity as follows:

(i) automatic respiration coincided with loss of consciousness;

(ii) the eyelid reflex, the swallowing reflex and the conjunctival reflexes disappeared in that order;

(iii) progressive depression of reflex activity of the intercostal and abdominal muscles, necessary for relaxation, was evident by reversal of normal respiratory rhythm, which, dependent only on the diaphragm, assumed a gasping character with the pause after *inspiration* instead of after expiration.

Many of these signs are absent when patients are anaesthetised by intravenous agents and paralysed by muscle relaxants. In these circumstances, the anaesthetist administers only enough anaesthetic, which, from experience with patients who do not receive relaxants, he knows is sufficient to maintain a light plane of anaesthesia, thus avoiding any possibility of overdose.

HOW LONG DOES IT TAKE TO RECOVER FROM AN ANAESTHETIC?

The speed of recovery depends on many factors, and can vary from a few minutes to half an hour or more.

Rapid recovery should occur after short operations and those where the anaesthetist has maintained a light plane of anaesthesia with inhalational agents like nitrous oxide, cyclopropane or halothane.

More prolonged recovery may follow very long procedures on debilitated patients.

A detailed chapter on recovery will be found on page 104.

2 PREPARATION OF THE PATIENT—I

PHYSICAL EXAMINATION AND ASSESSMENT

The object of pre-anaesthetic preparation is to make the patient *safe for surgery*. To this end, a member of the Anaesthetic Staff visits the patient as soon as the decision to operate has been taken. The purposes of this visit are: (i) to assess the patient's fitness to undergo anaesthesia and withstand the operation; (ii) to discover any defects in the physical state which may complicate the operation or recovery and arrange treatment to rectify these; (iii) to order pre-operative medication.

Pre-operative Assessment for Elective Surgery

After enquiring about general health and present illness, the anaesthetist undertakes a general physical examination of the patient paying particular attention to the *cardiovascular* and *respiratory system*, but not neglecting other factors to which the clinical history or symptoms draw attention, such as loss of weight, anaemia, dehydration or diabetes.

Examination of the Cardiovascular System

A normal blood-pressure, pulse rate, and exercise tolerance (capacity to negotiate stairs without undue breathlessness) suggest a normal cardiovascular system. A raised blood-pressure or a pulse which is rapid or irregular suggest an abnormality of the cardiovascular system, and further investigations will be necessary. The commonest abnormalities are: (i) valvular disease of the heart, (ii) coronary thrombosis, (iii) high blood-pressure and (iv) heart failure.

(i) *Valvular disease of the heart.* Rheumatic fever is a common cause of valvular disease, affecting the mitral valve between the right auricle and ventricle. If the patient is symptom free, this is no bar to operation. If signs of heart failure (see (iii)) are present or the pulse irregular (fibrillation), an electrocardiogram and the advice of a cardiologist may be required before deciding about fitness for the anaesthetic and operation.

(ii) *Coronary thrombosis.* A history of 'anginal pain' (attacks of severe pain in the chest which radiates down the arm) suggest the existence of coronary artery disease and the need for a diagnostic electrocardiogram. As this condition is often unsuspected by the patient an electrocardiogram is advisable for all patients over 60 before surgery. If there is evidence of previous coronary thrombosis and if it is known that the attack occurred within the past three months, the operation should be postponed (unless it is an emergency), since the operative mortality is increased within this period. After 3–4 months, recovery is considered to be complete so that surgery and anaesthesia do not constitute an additional hazard.

(iii) *Heart failure.* The signs and symptoms of heart failure: breathlessness at rest or on exertion; a fast and irregular pulse; distended neck veins are usually contra-indications to anaesthesia and require a period of rest and treatment with drugs such as digitalis before reassessment for fitness to undergo operation.

(iv) *High blood-pressure.* Excitement and apprehension frequently account for a high blood-pressure reading in patients newly admitted to hospital. Allowance should be made for this and if pressure is abnormally high in an otherwise healthy patient, a repeat of the observation 12 hours later, after administration of a calming dose of phenobarbitone will reveal a normal figure. *Hypertension*, (high blood-pressure) if properly controlled, does not constitute a bar to anaesthesia in the absence of heart failure or coronary arterial disease. In some instances, especially in the elderly, it is relatively benign and part of the natural processes of ageing.

If a patient is known to be under treatment for high blood-pressure, it is essential to know what drugs have been prescribed. Many drugs for this condition, although successful in controlling the complaint, can constitute an additional hazard during anaesthesia because many anaesthetics intensify their ability to lower blood-pressure (page 18).

Examination of the Respiratory System

Before examination of the chest, an enquiry should be made about smoking habits, the presence of early morning cough, and how much sputum is brought up. If the quantity is considerable, it should be collected and measured. The common cold and its aftermath of tracheal irritation and spasmodic cough is justification for postponing all but the most trivial or emergency operations for a few days, because the risk of post-operative chest infection (see below) is greatly increased.

After these preliminary investigations a full clinical examination of the chest is necessary. If this suggests the presence of impaired respiratory function, an X-ray of the chest and the performance of *Respiratory Function Tests* will indicate whether it is advisable to recommend a period of preparatory treatment aimed at improving the respiratory function before anaesthesia. Disorders of the respiratory tract; chronic bronchitis and emphysema, are a common cause of 'post-operative chests'. In patients who undergo abdominal operations (including hernias), the pain of the wound restricts breathing and expansion of the bases of the lungs. They also do not cough effectively enough to remove bronchial secretions, which accumulate in the deeper parts of the lungs, blocking the smaller bronchioles, so that the alveoli collapse (since no air reaches them) and patches of inflammation (broncho-pneumonia) develop. The risk of these complications can be much reduced by a few days of physiotherapy, supervised by a physiotherapist, assisted by the nursing staff. The measures adopted include:

(i) *Breathing exercises*. The patient is taught to expand the chest fully and is encouraged to cough and clear the chest of phlegm and sputum. This may be preceded by 'chest clapping'; (the palm of one hand is placed over the lower part of the chest, and a sharp blow given with the other hand) which loosens secretions in the deeper parts of the lung. This procedure may be necessary several times a day. Once the patient knows what is required to clear the chest, co-operation is more probable after the operation when the same procedure is continued for the first few days.

(ii) *Postural drainage*. Postural drainage is carried out when sputum is very copious. The patient lies in a head-down position with the affected side uppermost, so that accumulated secretions can drain into the main bronchus from whence expulsive coughing can remove them.

(iii) *No smoking*. Cigarette smoking aggravates cough and the production of sputum. If it can be established that giving up smoking can make a positive contribution to the success of the operation and to personal comfort, co-operation may be forthcoming.

(iv) *Inhalations* of isoprenaline or friar's balsam (tincture of benzoin) which dilate the bronchi and loosen sputum are an effective method of improving respiratory function.

Respiratory Function Tests

Complete assessment of respiratory function is a complicated procedure, carried out in the Cardio-Pulmonary Laboratory, and is restricted to patients who may require removal of one lung (pneumonectomy), or part of a lung (lobectomy). There are two simple tests which can be performed at the bedside without need for special apparatus: (1) *The match test.* Failure to blow out a lighted taper held six inches from the *open mouth* indicates impaired respiratory function and the need for further investigation. (2) *The breath-holding test.* Failure to hold the breath for 20 seconds also indicates either impaired respiratory or cardiac function.

The Vitalograph is a specially designed Spirometer for testing lung function which indicates the relevant findings in graphical form. It can be used at the bedside and explanation of the graphs helps the patient to understand why physiotherapy is necessary. After breathing exercises, and giving up smoking, function often improves and can be shown by improved graphs.

Anaemia and Blood Disorders

A full blood count, haemoglobin estimation, and blood grouping should be carried out before all major surgery. Haemoglobin values less than 10 mg per 100 ml (or 80%) are indications for treatment and possibly pre-operative blood transfusion. *Packed cells* (blood from which some plasma has been removed) are preferable to avoid overloading the circulation with excess fluid.

It is customary before all major procedures to order the cross-matching of a suitable amount of blood for transfusion during the operation.

Metabolic conditions: Diabetes

On admission to hospital urine should always be examined for albumin and sugar. If sugar is present, a test should be made for *acetone*. The presence of *acetone* is a danger signal because it indicates the presence of severe diabetes. If the condition is untreated, surgery and anaesthesia might precipitate *Diabetic coma*.

Diabetics under treatment require special preparation to ensure that sufficient glucose is given during the period before and after operation when no food can be taken by mouth, together with some reduction of the insulin dosage. The main danger is *Hypoglycaemic coma* from too little sugar in the blood, which could be a cause of delay in recovery.

The normal procedure on the day of operation is: (i) to change from Lente to Soluble Insulin, (ii) to replace breakfast with 500 mg of glucose given intravenously (500 ml of 5% Dextrose), (iii) to withhold insulin after operation until the blood sugar value has been obtained, (iv) the urine should be tested for *glucose* and *acetone* just before the patient leaves for the operating suite, and the result recorded on the operation sheet. If *acetone* is present, the anaesthetist must be told immediately. It indicates that the condition is out of control. Further treatment with intravenous glucose and insulin will be necessary before operation can proceed.

DRUGS CAUSING ADVERSE REACTIONS WITH ANAESTHETICS

There is a heading on many anaesthetic charts entitled 'drug history'. This is a reminder of the need to enquire for treatment with drugs which can induce dangerous reactions following pre-anaesthetic medication or during anaesthesia. Since such hazards have become more widely known many patients receiving such drugs are given a *drug card* by their pharmacist stating the name and dose of the drug, and with instructions to show it if admitted to hospital. Reliance cannot be placed on this procedure which does not replace the necessity to *enquire* about drugs in every instance. Often it is not practicable to stop administration before anaesthesia since the effects may persist for a week or more after withdrawal.

Three groups of drugs are of particular concern to anaesthetists. These are: 1. *Monoamine oxidase inhibitors* (M.A.O.I. drugs). 2. *Hypotensive drugs* (drugs for treatment of high blood-pressure). 3. *Steroids.*

(1) Monoamine oxidase inhibitors inhibit the action of an enzyme, monoamine oxidase, present in the liver, intestine, and brain which breaks down amines present in food (e.g. cheese) and those produced in the body—adrenaline and nor-adrenaline. Adverse reactions may follow administration of vaso-pressors (page 191), and pethidine (page 189). Since adrenaline is not destroyed, vaso-pressor drugs can induce very high blood-pressure followed by convulsions and coma. (Adrenaline in local anaesthetic solutions is not free from this hazard.) *Pethidine* may cause excitement; hyperthermia (high temperature) followed by convulsions and unconsciousness. Although similar responses might be expected to follow other opiates they have not so far been reported.

Monoamine oxidase inhibitors are: *iproniazid* ('Marsilid'), *isocarboxazid* ('Marplan'), *nialamide* ('Niamid'), *phenolzine* ('Nardil') and *tranylcypromine* ('Parnate').

(2) Drugs used for treatment of hypertension inhibit the *formation* of adrenaline and nor-adrenaline, or *block their action* on blood vessels. Anaesthetics (particularly intravenous barbiturates or halothane) also lower blood-pressure and when administered to patients being treated with this class of drugs, this is more pronounced. It is therefore essential to inform the anaesthetist if patients are receiving treatment for high blood-pressure so that he can modify his technique.

Hypotensive agents with adrenergic blocking actions are: *debrisoquine* ('Declinax'); *bethanidine* ('Esbatal'); *bretylium* ('Darenthin' and *guanethidine* ('Ismelin'). *Methyldopa* ('Aldomet') is an enzyme which prevents the formation of nor-adrenaline.

(3) Steroids are preparations of the secretion of the *adrenal cortex* which protect the body against the effects of infection and injury (known as 'stress'). They may be used in the treatment of chronic illnesses like *rheumatoid arthritis*, *ulcerative colitis*, *asthma* and certain *skin diseases*. Steroids depress the capacity of the adrenal cortex to produce cortisone in response to the 'stress' of infection; injury; anaesthesia and surgery. Patients under treatment with steroids require supplementary doses to avoid circulatory collapse during or following operation. Depression of adrenal function persists a considerable time after withdrawal of the drugs. If treatment has been given within *six months* of operation 100 mg cortisone acetate should be given the night before operation, and on the following morning. In emergency *hydrocortisone succinate* ('Neocortef') or *hydrocortisone di-sodium phosphate* ('Efcortesol') can be given intravenously prior to anaesthesia. One of these products should always be available during operation for treatment of any sudden collapse.

PRE-OPERATIVE ASSESSMENT FOR EMERGENCY SURGERY

Speed is the overriding consideration before emergency surgery. Apart from treatment of *shock*, *haemorrhage* or *dehydration*, the preparatory formalities are few.

Shocked patients. The presence of shock and/or haemorrhage is suggested by the presence of sweating; pallor; a thready pulse, and usually, but not invariably, a low blood-pressure. *Resuscitation* will be necessary before anaesthesia and consists of: (1) Relief of pain by opiates e.g. (Morphine or Pethidine). (2) *Intravenous Infusions* (saline, dextran or plasma) whilst a specimen of blood is being grouped and cross-matched with compatible blood. (3) *Warmth* by blankets.

A favourable response is indicated by: (1) The skin becoming warm and dry. (2) An improved *pulse volume* and decrease in pulse rate. (3) Rise in blood-pressure.

Dehydration is the result of loss of body fluids by: (1) Vomiting and diarrhoea. (2) Inability to drink from weakness. (3) Excessive secretion of fluid into the bowel (such as occurs following intestinal obstruction) or into the cavity of the abdomen from peritonitis (inflammation of the peritoneum) after perforation of stomach or bowel.

The signs of dehydration are: (1) Dry and inelastic skin—for example, after pinching the skin of the forearm, it remains puckered and does not resume its normal shape. (2) A dry tongue, pointed nose and sunken eyes ('Hippocratic Facies'). (3) Rapid, thready pulse and low blood-pressure.

Treatment of dehydration. (1) *Intravenous Fluids*—e.g. glucose saline (page 81)—considerable quantities may be necessary. The main deficiency is usually *sodium* and *chloride*. *Examination of blood for electrolyte levels* is essential at the beginning and at subsequent intervals to assess the results of treatment.

(2) *Passage of a naso-gastric tube* and aspiration of stomach contents every 15 minutes (recording the amount and nature of the aspirated fluid and retaining it for inspection). Yellow, light or dirty brown, foul-smelling fluid is a finding in intestinal obstruction.

Known colloquially as 'Drip and Suction', this form of treatment continues until the patient's deficit of water and salts has been restored. This is judged partly by improvement in the clinical condition (moist tongue, reduced pulse rate and improved volume) and partly by return towards normal of the electrolyte contents of the blood as shown by chemical analysis. The time taken may last several hours, but the reduced mortality which results justifies the delay.

3 PREPARATION OF THE PATIENT—II

PRE-ANAESTHETIC MEDICATION AND TRANSFER TO THE OPERATING SUITE

The objects of pre-anaesthetic medication are to allay the fear of the operation; to produce a calm and well-rested patient on the day of operation, and to minimise as far as possible the hazards of anaesthesia and surgery. It is *partly psychological* and *partly prophylactic*.

In order to 'produce a calm well-rested patient on the day of operation' something more than the customary hypodermic injection an hour before operation is often necessary; in fact pre-anaesthetic medication can usefully begin at the time of admission to hospital. In the interval that elapses between arrival in hospital and the day of operation all patients receive the routine examination already described, whilst many undergo additional investigations and preparatory measures. These can often accentuate an uneasiness whose origin is separation from family or business responsibilities. Men worry about their job or their office affairs whilst women become anxious about the well-being of their family. Many patients find adaptation to a strange environment difficult. Hospital 'smells' nauseate some patients whilst others find the lack of privacy in a public ward embarrassing. Fear of the impending anaesthetic is universal and often exceeds that of the operation itself. Whilst many express their feelings freely, others may try to conceal them beneath an outward show of bravado and forced heartiness.

Sympathy and kindness can do much to dispel such fears, and nurses, by virtue of their closer contact with the patient, can help greatly in this respect. If, in spite of these efforts, patients remain tense and anxious, drugs may be prescribed to calm the mind and ensure adequate sleep. *Tranquillisers* and *hypnotics* are useful in such circumstances.

Tranquillisers induce a calm state of mind without sleepiness and are sometimes called 'day-time sedatives': examples are, chlordiazepoxide ('Librium'), diazepam ('Valium'), or hydroxyzine ('Atarax' or 'Vistaril').

Hypnotics are colloquially known as 'sleeping pills'. Most patients need a hypnotic when in hospital because sound sleep is difficult to achieve in strange surroundings and the disturbance from ward activity at night which cannot always be avoided. *Barbiturate preparations* are most commonly used for this purpose although non-barbiturates are also very effective (see p. 186).

The Pre-operative Injection ('Premedication')

One hour before the scheduled time of the operation an injection is given traditionally consisting of an **opiate** (p. 183) together with atropine or hyoscine ('Scopolamine'). The opiate replaces anxiety by a carefree state of mind (euphoria), but since some patients are depressed and nauseated by opiates, a hypnotic, or tranquilliser may be substituted.

Atropine (p. 184) depresses vagus activity during anaesthesia which would be evident as (*a*) excessive secretion of saliva and mucus in the respiratory tract, and (*b*) slowing of the heart (bradycardia) with a risk of cardiac arrest especially during induction of anaesthesia or endotracheal intubation. Atropine dries up secretions (causes dryness of the mouth) and increases the pulse rate and thus avoids these responses.

Hyoscine ('Scopolamine'), in addition to a 'drying' action like atropine, also has an 'amnesic' effect, so that there is little or no recollection of events taking place whilst under its influence.

Major tranquillisers (p. 190) may also be included in the pre-anaesthetic injection. **Phenothiazines**, e.g. Promethazine ('Phenergan') (p. 189), intensify the action of opiates, Promazine ('Sparine'), Chlorpromazine ('Largactil') reduce nausea and vomiting and calm the mind. **Butyrophenones** (e.g. 'Droperidol') (p. 184) are especially effective in induction of a state of complete indifference, before procedures under local or regional anaesthesia.

Some well-known pre-operative injections are:

(*a*) **Papaveretum** ('Omnopon') 20 mg and **Hyoscine** 0·4 mg
(*b*) **Pethidine** (Demerol, Meperidine) 100 mg. **Atropine** 0·6 mg
(*c*) **Morphine** 10–15 mg and **Atropine** 0·6 mg
(*d*) **Pethidine** 100 mg and **Promethazine** 50 mg ('Pamergan' P. 100)

Dosage varies with the age and physical state of the patient. For very old patients, opiates are now usually replaced by Diazepam orally or intravenously together with Atropine.

Note. All pre-operative injections except **papaveretum** ('Omnopon') and **morphine** and **atropine** should be given by the intramuscular route. Special care should be taken when injecting promethazine ('Phenergan') and other phenothiazines (p. 190) to avoid placing the injection in the proximity of a nerve since they possess local anaesthetic properties which can cause permanent damage to nerves.

Timing of the pre-operative injection

Nursing staff often worry about the time the pre-operative injection should be given. Usually it is ordered one hour before operation, but this can be difficult to assess with certainty unless the patient happens to be first on the list. It is better to give it *too soon than too late* because it is effective within half an hour, and the effect lasts for several hours. Since its main purpose is to induce sleep, the patient, hungry and often thirsty, benefits; his time of waiting become less burdensome, whilst the protective action is by no means lessened.

Sometimes, owing to changes in the order of operating, the injection may not have been given when the call comes from the theatre. It is pointless to delay things in order to give the injection as there will be no time for it to become effective. The pre-operative injection can be given intravenously together with, or before, induction of anaesthesia. Although the patient is denied the calming effect of the injection, if there is no delay in the anaesthetic room, anxiety is reduced to a minimum.

PREPARATION OF CHILDREN

Children require special consideration.

Infants (under 2 years) have little or no recollection of an anaesthetic.

Older children (3–7 years) are more perceptive and imaginative. Removal from parents and familiar surroundings induces a feeling of insecurity. Every effort should be made to obtain their trust and confidence. It is better to treat them as an equal and explain in simple terms what is happening. *The parents* are often more anxious and their feelings may find expression in excessive fussing and reluctance to leave the child. Children often sense the anxiety of their parents which they reflect in their own behaviour. In such circumstances, it is helpful to concentrate on getting to know the parents and discovering a child's peculiarities and attitudes, which will be of great help in making him feel at ease when the parents are absent. If a child is subnormal, e.g. spastic or mongoloid, the mother should be allowed to remain with the child throughout its stay in hospital.

If a child does not settle after the departure of its parents but remains tearful and miserable, a tranquilliser e.g. hydroxyzine will induce calm and help adjustment to the new environment.

Pre-anaesthetic Medication

Although the drugs used for adult premedication are suitable for children in *reduced* amounts, there are certain differences in emphasis and approach:

The *oral* and *rectal* routes of administration are more often used. Children, especially below the age of 7–8, dislike injections. Some will burst into tears at the sight of a hypodermic syringe. Sweet syrupy preparations are prepared to disguise the bitter and acid taste of most drugs. An alternative is to mix them with honey or jam.

Dosage is calculated according to the weight of the child. This information should be available.

Anaesthetists differ in their attitudes towards pre-operative medication. Some prefer atropine only, and rely on the co-operation of the child at induction in the interests of a rapid recovery. Others favour hypnotics and/or tranquillisers in order to reduce psychic trauma. Often the decision depends on the temperament of the child, whether excitable and imaginative or calm and phlegmatic.

For this reason, a detailed discussion of premedicant drugs would not be profitable. The following are some of the common drugs used:

(i) **Atropine**. The dose from the age of 2 onwards is the same as the adult dose. Children tolerate this drug well—except in *hot weather* or when *febrile*, when its property of *preventing sweating* can cause *hyperpyrexia* (high temperature and convulsions).

(ii) *Tranquillisers.* **Promethazine** ('Phenergan') and **trimeprazine** ('Vallergan') are available in syrupy form known as 'Elixir'. The dosage is relatively large (promethazine 1 mg/kg, trimeprazine 2 mg/kg). They may be prescribed *alone* for their calming effect or with barbiturates to induce sleep.

(iii) *Barbiturates.* Dosage 0·5 mg per year of age up to a maximum of 1·5 mg given by the *oral route.* Most children fall asleep if left alone in quiet surroundings.

(iv) The combinations of **papaveretum** ('Omnopon') or **pethidine** with **atropine**, **hyoscine** or **promethazine** which adults receive are suitable for children, but in dosage calculated according to their weight (Table 1).

When the pre-anaesthetic medication has been given, the child's attention should be diverted from his immediate surroundings by screens (if in an open ward) and, if old enough, by reading a story until he falls asleep. The transfer to the theatre trolley will arouse him but if comfortably wrapped in warm blankets a short pause will allow the return of sleep before proceeding. Conversation is unnecessary unless the child awakes when he should be encouraged to fall asleep again.

TABLE 1

Scale of dosage of Papaveretum and Hyoscine for Children

Weight (kg)	Papaveretum (mg)	Hyoscine (mg)
13–20	6	0·1
20–25	10	0·2
25–30	15	0·3
30 and over	20	0·4

(v) *Rectal premedication.* **Thiopentone** 40 mg/kg body weight, to a maximum of 2 g, dissolved in 20 ml water administered rectally 30–40 minutes before operation is a certain method of making sure the child is in a deep sleep before leaving his ward with no recollection of the anaesthetic. Timing is important as the effects pass off within one hour.

(vi) **Ketalar** can be given intramuscularly to small children under 3 years of age when difficulties arise with parents or the child is unduly disturbed.

FINAL PREPARATIONS ON THE DAY OF OPERATION

On the day of operation there are a number of final preparations to be observed. These concern the following: (1) Ensuring that the patient's *stomach is empty*. (2) The signature of a *form of consent* for the operation and anaesthetic. (3) *Removal of dentures*, jewellery and other valuables. (4) *Checking, administration and recording* of the pre-anaesthetic injection. (5) Assembly of the patient's notes and X-rays. (6) Checking on availability of blood for transfusion. (7) Communication with the operating theatre.

(1) The importance of an empty stomach. The presence of food in the stomach increases the hazard of inhalation of stomach contents into the air passages, either from regurgitation into the pharynx during the operation or from vomiting during induction or recovery.

The patient should neither eat nor drink on the day of operation, unless it is not scheduled to take place until late in the afternoon when a light breakfast of sweet tea and toast before 8 a.m. is permissible.

Before anaesthesia for *emergency procedures* enquiries should be made when the last meal was taken and of what it consisted. Normally the stomach empties in 3 to 4 hours. After accidents *there is delay in emptying of up to 6 hours.* If food or drink has recently been taken it may be necessary to empty the stomach with a stomach tube.

(2) Consent forms. The form of consent should have been signed before the day of operation. Whoever is responsible for the final preparations should make a check about this and see that it is included in the patient's notes. The Family Law Reform Act of 1969, which implements the decision to reduce the coming of age from 21 to 18 years, also includes a section which states that any person of 16 years upwards may sign a consent form, thus removing some confusion which has existed about this in the past. There are also circumstances, for example in emergency, when persons under sixteen may sign a consent form if they have sufficient mental capacity to know what the consent implies.

(3) Removal of dentures and valuables. (*a*) *Dentures.* All dentures should be removed after the pre-anaesthetic injection because, if displaced during induction of anaesthesia, they can cause respiratory obstruction. Small dentures are especially dangerous. It is not enough to *ask* about dentures. It is better to look in the mouth. Some patients are forgetful and others too embarrassed to admit owning dentures. (*b*) Rings, watches or other jewellery should be removed and handed to the ward sister for safe keeping.

(4) The pre-anaesthetic injection (p. 23). The checking of the pre-anaesthetic medication before administration is a normal nursing routine. Attention should be given to whether it is to be given by the intramuscular or subcutaneous routes. The purpose of the injection should be explained to the patient who, when it has been given, should lie *flat* with one pillow, be screened from the other patients, and encouraged to sleep. The details should be entered and signed on the Anaesthetic Sheet or Operation Record.

(5) Assembly of patient's notes and X-rays. All the clinical notes and X-rays belonging to the patient should be assembled ready by the bedside for transfer with the patient to the operating suite.

(6) Checking of availability of blood. Not all patients will require a blood transfusion during the operation, but if reference to the patient's clinical records shows there has been a request for blood it is advisable to check that the blood is *ready* and available. Cross matching takes several hours and in emergency there will be some delay. The anaesthetist will appreciate information about this.

(7) Communication with the operating suite. Every hospital has a system to ensure that the correct patient goes to the correct theatre. Unless there is a standard procedure mistakes can happen, especially when more than one operating theatre is in use. The following procedure is an example:

When the theatre is ready for the patient the theatre superintendent sends an orderly to the ward with the slip of paper on which is written:

(*a*) The ward, name, and hospital number of the patient.
(*b*) The nature of the proposed operation.

On receiving this slip the sister or nurse in charge of the ward checks this against the theatre operating list, the patient's notes and identity band. If satisfied that all agree she arranges for a nurse to accompany the patient. Before leaving, the nurse should once more check on the points already mentioned. The procedure to be followed on arrival at the anaesthetic room is discussed on page 94.

PREPARATION OF DAY PATIENTS

Day patients are admitted to hospital in the morning for an examination or operation during the day and return home in the evening. This practice is growing in popularity, especially in areas where demand for surgical beds is high and waiting lists are long.

Preparation for anaesthesia, and after-care, follow the principles already laid down, but as the time available is limited it is important that procedure in any particular hospital should be clearly defined. Mutual understanding with the family doctor and close co-operation between the surgical and anaesthetic teams are essential for the success of the scheme from the moment the procedure is arranged in the out-patient clinic, until discharge from hospital.

Selection of Day Patients

Conditions suitable for day treatment include (*a*) *Diagnostic Examinations* e.g. cystoscopy, bronchoscopy, sigmoidoscopy and certain radiological examinations. (*b*) *Orthopaedic procedures*, manipulations, reduction of fractures, change of plaster and certain minor operative procedures. (*c*) *General surgical and gynaecological operations*, from those of a minor nature—removal of cysts; dilatation and curettage, to relatively major undertakings such as hernioplasty and operations on varicose veins.

Only those who are in apparently good health, under 60 and with home conditions suitable for adequate after-care are chosen as day patients. Once agreement has been obtained and a consent form signed (usually in the out-patient clinic), preliminary assessment of fitness to undergo the procedure under general or local anaesthetic should be undertaken.

An appointment should be made for a member of the anaesthetic staff to see the patient (some hospitals hold out-patient clinics for this purpose). If this cannot be done immediately the following examinations can be conveniently undertaken.

(1) *X-ray of chest* (to exclude pulmonary disease).
(2) *Red cell count* and *haemoglobin estimation* (to exclude anaemia).
(3) *Urine test* for albumin and sugar (to exclude urinary disease or diabetes).
(4) If the patient is over 50—an *electrocardiographic examination*. (To avoid undue pressure on the E.C.G. Department this might be left to the discretion of the anaesthetist.)

The findings of the above examinations and any other relevant information should be carefully recorded in the patient's notes.

Every patient should receive a card of general instructions which should include the absolute necessity (for his own safety) of abstaining from food or drink on the day of operation.

Procedure on the day of operation (day patients)

On arrival at hospital, as soon as the patient is in bed, a member of the anaesthetic staff should be called. On arrival he will carry out such examinations as he thinks necessary (dependent on the finding of the preparatory examinations already noted) and prescribe a pre-operation injection. *Both anaesthetic and nursing staff should satisfy themselves by direct questioning that the patient has complied with the instructions concerning food and drink.* From this point, procedure before anaesthesia does not differ from that for in-patients.

Note. The nursing staff should not fail to ensure that a consent form has been signed.

Recovery

Normal recovery room routine follows the anaesthetic. Since the technique chosen should be one ensuring a rapid return of consciousness no undue delay in return to the ward should occur at this stage.

Post-operative pain or discomfort may require injection of an analgesic after some procedures, but for the majority an oral analgesic such as paracetamol, or codeine compound (pp. 185, 189) will be adequate. Nausea can be relieved by oral anti-emetics (p. 184).

Discharge and Return Home

Soon after return to the ward the patient should be ready to take some light refreshment e.g. sweet tea or coffee and dry biscuits.

Before discharge the surgeon and anaesthetist should see the patient. The surgeon is concerned with the wound—security of the dressing and absence of bleeding. The anaesthetist must be satisfied that the patient is not only *conscious* but that his *cerebral condition is normal*. Speech should not be slurred, and full awareness of the day of the week, of the surroundings, and of the need for care of the wound should be demonstrable. He should give an undertaking not to attempt to drive a car, or any other conveyance for 24 hours.

After general anaesthesia a patient should never leave the hospital unaccompanied. Before leaving he should be given (*a*) written instructions about after-care and the signs and symptoms of any possible complications together with clear instructions to contact the hospital or his general practitioner should they occur. (*b*) A supply of drugs to ensure sleep and control pain or discomfort.

4 THE ANAESTHETIC ROOM—I

The anaesthetic room is a small room between the operating theatre and the main corridor of the suite. It is designed to provide: (i) a place where the patient can be taken on arrival at the operating suite and be spared the sight and the sounds of the preparations for the operation; (ii) the opportunity to induce anaesthesia undisturbed by the noise and movement of the rest of the surgical team and (iii) a storage place for apparatus and equipment.

The decoration of the room differs from the rest of the suite in an attempt to conceal its clinical purpose. Diffuse ceiling lighting spares the eyes of a patient lying on a trolley. Soft pastel colours on the walls and decorated ceilings represent an attempt to deflect the thoughts of the conscious patient from the business in hand.

CONTROL OF ACCESS TO THE ANAESTHETIC ROOM

Access to the anaesthetic room should be restricted to anaesthetic staff at all times and not only when the patient is waiting induction, to prevent its use as a short cut between theatre and the main corridor.

CONTENTS OF THE ANAESTHETIC ROOM

The fixed furnishings of the anaesthetic room consist of: (i) cupboards, which contain drugs, equipment and stocks of intravenous fluids; (ii) a washhand basin; a sink and worktop for preparation of equipment and drugs; (iii) a spot light suspended from the ceiling or wall for use when making an intravenous puncture.

Movable equipment consists of the anaesthetic machine; ventilator; drip stand; monitoring apparatus, and a dressing trolley for equipment which may be needed in the theatre. In American hospitals where the operating suite may contain as many as twenty operating theatres (operating rooms) the anaesthetic room contains no fixed equipment. Everything the anaesthetist needs comes from a central store on trolleys. In other American hospitals anaesthetic rooms are not provided and anaesthesia is induced in the operating room. This is not as terrifying as it may appear, because no sterilisation of instruments takes place in the operating area. Pre-packed instruments are laid out and covered with a towel before the patient arrives in the operating room, which by that time differs little in appearance from an anaesthetic room.

A nurse or technician should be responsible for the tidiness of the anaesthetic room and for the preliminary preparations for anaesthesia before the arrival of the patient. This requires a knowledge of the contents of the anaesthetic room which the remainder of this and subsequent chapters aim to provide.

ANAESTHETIC APPARATUS

The standard apparatus (Boyle's) consists of a square-topped *metal trolley* with racks for *gas cylinders* around the sides, and a bracket at the back which carries *flowmeters* to measure the flow of gases and *vaporisers* (glass bottles or metal containers) for liquid anaesthetics (Fig. 6). The top of the trolley accommodates small items of equipment like airways, syringes and drugs. At the bottom there is a drawer in which the blood pressure cuff, spare airways and record cards may be kept. The space between the top of the trolley and the drawer is clear but may house a *carbon dioxide absorption apparatus* (page 46) or *ventilator* (Chapter 15). A corrugated rubber tube and reservoir bag attached to the right hand side of the bracket conveys the anaesthetic to the patient.

The Gas Cylinders. Gas cylinders are coloured in accordance with an international code to prevent confusion in identification. A card showing colours of all gas cylinders should be displayed on the wall of the anaesthetic room. Where anaesthetic rooms are not equipped with piped gases, there are six cylinders on the anaesthetic machine: two of *Nitrous oxide* (international colour *blue*); two of *Oxygen* (international colour *black* with *white* shoulders); one of *Carbon dioxide* (international colour *grey*); one of *Cyclopropane* (international colour *orange*). The cyclopropane cylinder is attached to a bracket yoke at the left-hand side of the front of the trolley.

There are *two* cylinders of *nitrous oxide* because, being a weak anaesthetic it is used in large quantities. Should a cylinder become empty during an operation it would be difficult to keep the patient anaesthetised unless it was possible for change to a full one immediately.

When the operating suite is equipped with piped gases, one cylinder of oxygen and one of nitrous oxide remain for use should the piped supply fail.

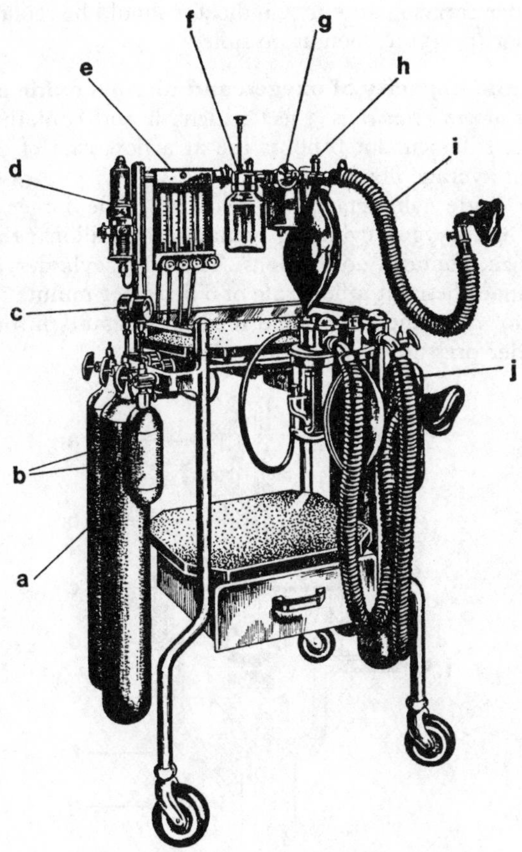

Fig. 6 Standard Boyle's apparatus

a cyclopropane cylinder
b oxygen cylinder
c pressure gauges
d Bosun warning device
e rotameters
f ether vaporiser
g fluothane vaporiser
h emergency oxygen tap
i Magill attachment
j circle absorber unit and tubes

Carbon dioxide is used to stimulate respiration during inhalational induction or to restore carbon dioxide to the blood after a period of over-breathing (hyperventilation with a mechanical ventilator), or after anaesthesia with carbon dioxide absorption.

Indicator Discs. Metal indicator discs show which cylinder is FULL and which is IN USE. A third one marked EMPTY replaces the IN USE indicator when a cylinder becomes exhausted whilst the FULL indicator on the fresh cylinder is replaced by one marked IN USE.

A cylinder carrying an EMPTY indicator should be replaced with a full cylinder (p. 35) as soon as possible.

Size and capacity of oxygen and nitrous oxide cylinders. *A standard oxygen cylinder* is 3 feet in length and contains 24 cubic feet of gas, sufficient for 6 hours use at a flow rate of 2 litres per minute (an average flow).

Nitrous oxide cylinders are of two sizes. The larger (the same length as the oxygen cylinder) contains 400 gallons; the smaller, half the size, contains 200 gallons. The large cylinder provides 6 hours of anaesthesia at a flow rate of 6 litres per minute (often used in practice). Note the use of fluid measure because nitrous oxide is stored under pressure in liquid form (p. 35).

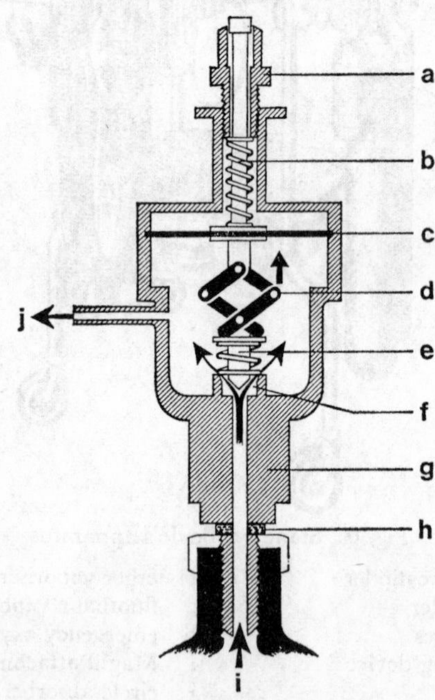

Fig. 7 The principle and mechanism of a reducing valve

a adjustable screw cap
b spring surrounding metal rod
c diaphragm
d toggle
e valve
f gas inlet
g central metal cone
h fibre washer
i gas from cylinder
j gas outlet (7 lb/in^2)

One *full* cylinder of *nitrous oxide* and one *full oxygen* cylinder supplies oxygen and nitrous oxide for more than 6 hours of anaesthesia. When carbon-dioxide absorption is in use (p. 46) reduced flow rates are possible and cylinder life considerably prolonged.

Reducing Valves. Each cylinder is fitted with a *pressure-reducing valve* to reduce the pressure of gas emerging from *2,000 pounds* per square inch in *oxygen* cylinders, and *750 pounds* per square inch in *nitrous oxide* cylinders to between *7 and 10 pounds* per square inch. Its purpose is to protect the patient and allow accurate control of the flow of gases.

A reducing valve (Fig. 7) consists of a central metal core whose lower end connects with the gas supply, and whose upper part expands into a metal cylinder containing the pressure reducing mechanism. This consists of a metal rod pressed down by a strong spring. The gas pressure must overcome the resistance of the spring in order to lift the end of the rod sealing the channel to the cylinder and emerge from the supply tube on the side of the valve. A screw at the top of the valve when turned *clockwise* increases the tension on the spring, reducing the pressure of the emerging gas. Turning in the reverse direction increases the pressure.

To simplify identification, each valve carries a coloured disc on its upper surface, identical with the international code with the name of the gas in black lettering.

Pin Index Safety System. The Pin Index Safety System is an international standard device designed to make quite certain that the wrong cylinder can *never* be connected to the wrong valve. Each reducing valve carries two small pins placed in such a manner that they will only fit into correspondingly spaced holes on the neck of the cylinder for which it is intended (Fig. 8). (Some years ago a popular thriller illustrated the need for this device. Titled 'Green for Danger', it concerned the murder of a patient under anaesthesia by connecting a carbon dioxide cylinder—coloured green in those days —to the oxygen valve, so that the patient died of carbon dioxide poisoning before the anaesthetist discovered the mistake.) This would have been impossible with the Pin Index System.

Pressure Indicator Gauges. Oxygen cylinder valves carry a small circular watch type dial which records the *pressure* (and quantity) of gas in the cylinder. As the oxygen is used pressure indicated by the needle falls gradually to zero thus showing the cylinder is empty. Nitrous oxide valves do not usually carry pressure gauges because they give no indication of the quantity of gas in the cylinder. Nitrous oxide exists in liquid form in the cylinder, the quantity always being expressed in gallons. Since the pressure at the surface of a liquid is always constant, the pressure in the nitrous oxide cylinder will be unchanged until all the liquid has turned to gas, so a pressure indicator would continue to show a *full* cylinder until it was practically empty (Fig. 9). Weight is the only reliable

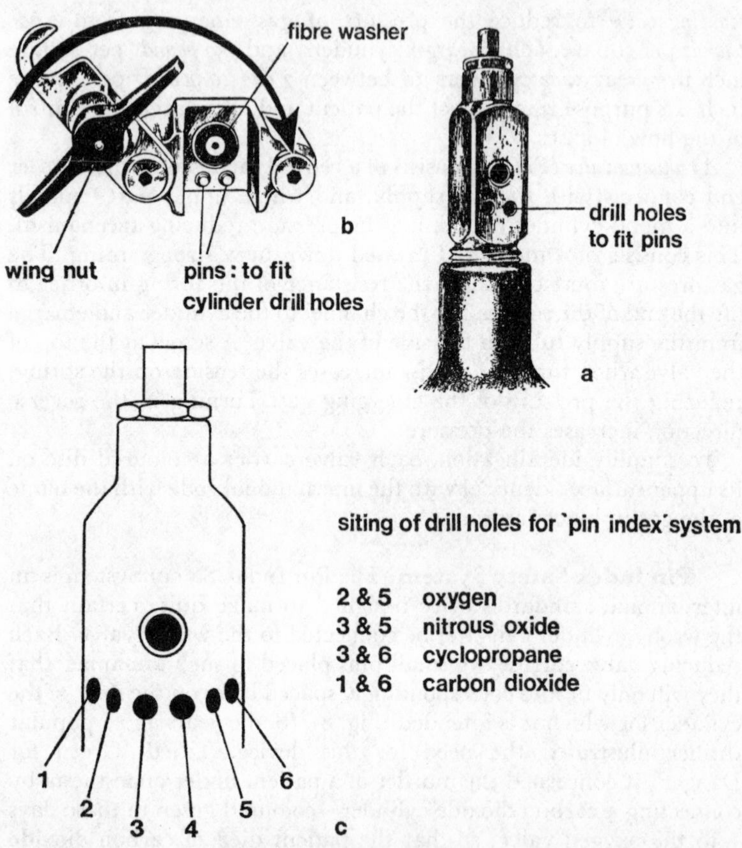

Fig. 8 Pin-index safety system

guide to the exact quantity of nitrous oxide. Every cylinder has figures stamped on its neck which indicate the weight when empty and when full, so that when in doubt one could weigh it. In practice this is never necessary because when a cylinder is filled a *red cellophane band is placed round the neck*, to distinguish it from an empty cylinder. *The band should not be removed until the cylinder is put into use* on the anaesthetic apparatus. *Cyclopropane*, being in liquid form also requires no pressure gauge.

Changing Cylinders. Before removing an 'empty' cylinder a replacement *with the red cellophane wrapper intact* should be ready.

The empty cylinder is removed by loosening the thumbscrew which keeps it in place; or (on older apparatus) by loosening the nut at the base of the reducing valve with a spanner. Care should be taken to ensure that a small fibre washer on the outlet of the valve does not fall off (Fig. 8). This washer ensures a leakproof junction between cylinder and valve. If worn or frayed it should be changed and replaced by a new one. A supply of washers should be kept in the drawer at the bottom of the trolley.

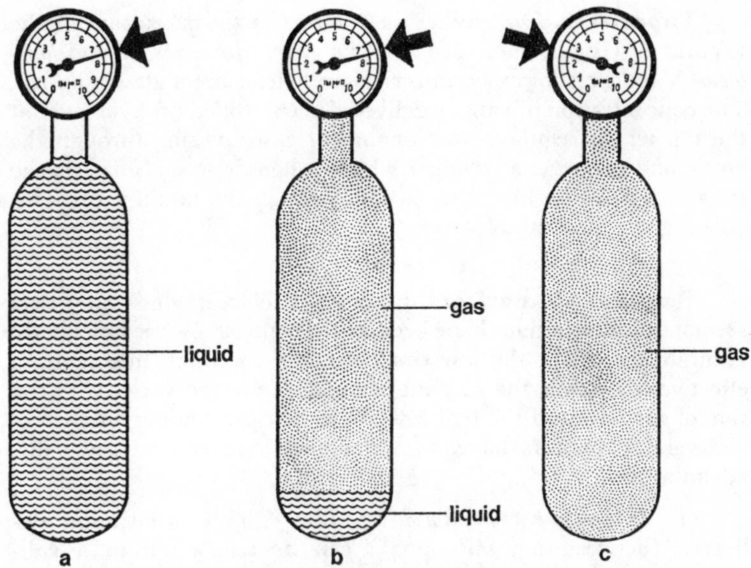

Fig. 9 Pressure indicator gauges with nitrous oxide

a cylinder, full pressure 750 lb/in²
b cylinder nearly empty, liquid present, pressure 750 lb/in²
c cylinder contains gas only, pressure falling

Having fixed the cylinder and tightened the screws which hold it in position the valve should be opened for a moment to make sure that there is no leak. A hissing sound indicates that gas is escaping and that there is need for tightening the screw, or if this fails, replacement of the fibre washer.

The Rotameters. The Rotameter Unit (Fig. 6) consists of a metal frame enclosing a series of vertical transparent tubes (one for each type of gas on the machine) graduated in litres and cubic centimetres. A screw valve at the base of the unit controls the flow of gas in each tube, and when opened the flow of gas pushes before it a small duralumin bobbin which executes a spinning movement (Rotameter) whilst allowing the gas to pass on. The figure on the tube level with the top of the bobbin indicates the rate of flow, in litres per minute.

Vaporisers. On leaving the rotameters the gases pass to the vaporisers. Usually there are *three*: for *ether*, *trichlorethylene* and *halothane*. Vaporisers for ether and trichlorethylene are of glass (Fig. 10). The concentration of vapour delivered is controlled (*a*) by a lever at the top which regulates the amount of gases passing through the bottle and (*b*) a metal plunger which, when depressed, directs the stream of gases on to the surface or through the liquid greatly increasing the quantity of vapour.

Halothane Vaporisers. Ether and trichlorethylene vaporisers are not suitable for halothane because the controls are not sufficiently accurate to deliver the low concentrations in which this agent is effective, moreover the amount of vapour delivered varies with the rate of gas flow and the temperature of the surrounding air.

Several vaporisers have been designed to overcome these disadvantages:

(1) *Temperature compensated vaporisers.* The concentration delivered (between 0·5 and 4·0%) can be selected from a calibrated control. The percentage in the mixture delivered is constant and independent of the temperature; the amount of liquid; or rate of gas flow. Well-known models are the 'Fluotec' (Fig. 10a) and the 'M.I.E. Temperature Compensated Vaporiser'. Both are of metal, with a concentration control at the top and a filling port at the lower end. The vaporiser can be filled by removing the screw plug from the filling port and pouring liquid in until the level in small window to the left of the port reaches the 'full' line.

(2) *The Goldman Inhaler* (Fig. 10a) is a simpler device consisting of a small glass chamber the size of an egg cup held in position by a metal clip and screw. A lever at the upper part controls the flow of gases. The concentration of vapour which it delivers cannot exceed 2% irrespective of the total gas flow. Metal inlet and outlets allow the unit to be inserted into any continuous gas flow apparatus.

Although originally designed for use with dental anaesthetic apparatus the vaporiser is also used on continuous flow machines, either alongside the other vaporisers or plugged into the inspiratory side of a carbon dioxide absorption unit. This latter position, known as 'vaporiser in circuit' (V.I.C.) is used by some anaesthetists to obtain high concentrations of halothane economically using low oxygen flow and complete re-breathing. The vaporiser should always be removed from this position after use.

Emergency oxygen supply. All apparatus carry an emergency oxygen tap. In many it is placed at the extreme right of the bracket carrying the flowmeters and vaporisers. It is connected directly to the oxygen cylinders, and delivers pure oxygen under slight pressure.

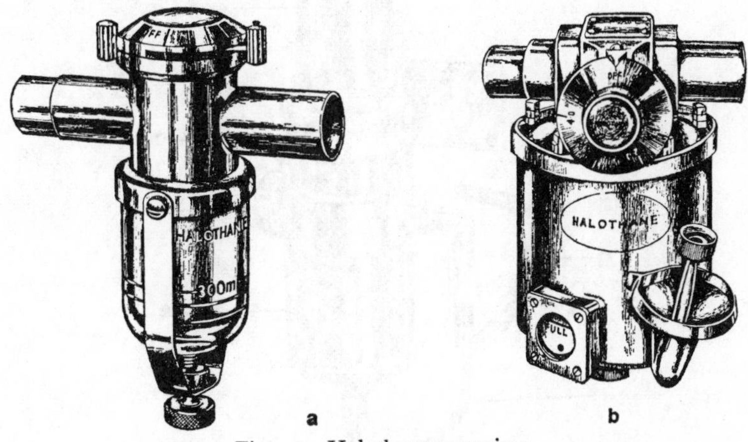

Fig. 10 Halothane vaporiser

a Goldman b Temperature condensed

The Bosun Warning Device. The Bosun Warning Device gives warning signals of the failure of oxygen supply by means of a whistle and red light (Fig. 11). It consists of a cylinder about 20 centimetres in length which is fixed by a bracket at the left-hand end of the anaesthetic trolley. The *upper part* of the cylinder is of metal and contains a 1·5 volt battery and small light bulb which illuminates a translucent red dome on the top of the cylinder. The *lower part* is transparent, containing a metal bellows connected to the oxygen supply by a small tube which emerges from its lower end. Between upper and lower cylinders there is a whistle connected to the nitrous oxide supply by a piece of metal tubing. A switch in the middle of the cylinder controls the light. (Older models also included a whistle control.)

How the Bosun works. When the oxygen cylinder is opened the gas pressure expands the metal bellows *breaking the contact* between the bulb and the battery and *closing the valve on the whistle* operated by nitrous oxide. When the *oxygen supply fails*, *pressure falls*, so that the bellows collapses *restoring contact between the battery and bulb* and the *red light* becomes visible, at the same time the *valve controlling nitrous oxide* opens and the *whistle sounds*.

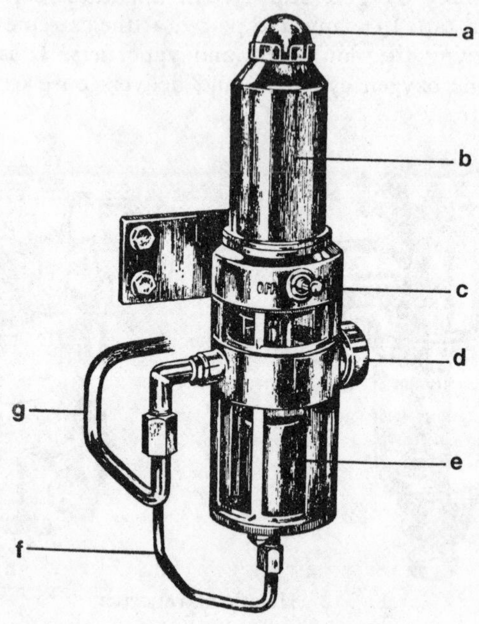

Fig. 11 Bosun Warning Device

a	red light	d	whistle	f	to oxygen supply
b	battery	e	metal bellows	g	to nitrous oxide supply
c	light control switch				

The red light and whistle are independent of each other for two reasons:

(1) *The whistle depends on the nitrous oxide.* Nitrous oxide may not always be used because oxygen alone is sufficient when administering halothane or cyclopropane. In these circumstances the whistle will not sound when the oxygen supply fails unless nitrous oxide cylinders are opened.

(2) *Should nitrous oxide fail at the same time as oxygen, the whistle will not operate, but the red light will still appear.* The chances of this occurrence may appear remote, but it is worth noting that used at customary flow rates the large cylinders containing 400 gallons of nitrous

oxide and 24 cubic feet of oxygen last about 6 hours, and thus could and do become 'empty' at the same time.

Testing the Bosun. The Bosun should always be tested at the beginning of the day's work. *To test red light and whistle*: (1) *Both*

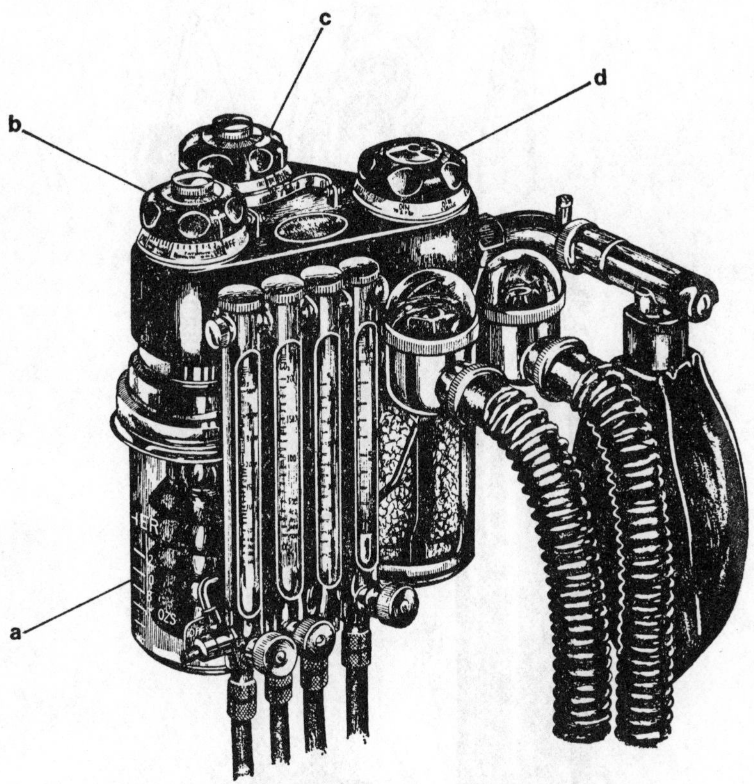

Fig. 12 The Marrett Head

a ether or halothane
b filling caps
c trichloroethylene
d absorber control

switches should be turned to the ON *position.* (2) *The nitrous oxide tap* should be opened, *leaving the oxygen closed*, and the oxygen tap opened to remove any oxygen from the tubing when the *red light* should appear and the *whistle* should sound.

To test the red light only. After closing all cylinders the flow-meter taps are opened to allow gases in the circuit to run off. When the oxygen rotameter falls to zero the *red light should appear*.

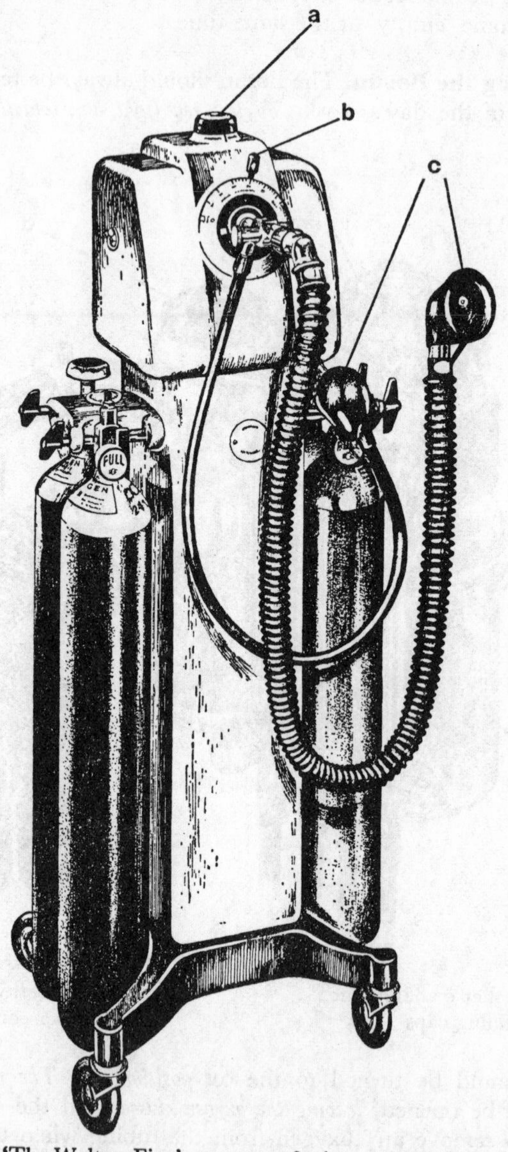

Fig. 13 'The Walton Five' apparatus for intermittent flow of gases

a pressure control b gas mixture control

c nasal attachment and facepiece

An improvement on the Bosun known as 'the oxygen failure warning device' will shortly become available. The signal of oxygen failure is a low pitched whistle and simultaneously the nitrous oxide flow is directed away from the patient in order to discontinue the anaesthetic.

OTHER TYPES OF ANAESTHETIC APPARATUS

The Marrett apparatus. The Marrett anaesthetic apparatus (Fig. 12) is a more compact assembly than the Boyle's. Any inhalational technique can be used without need for separate attachments, and continuous flow and absorption by 'Circle' or 'To and Fro' methods are all available. The Marrett 'head' is placed at the top of a stand carrying cylinders, and consists of three circular containers; one for ether, one for trichlorethylene, and one for soda lime, with rotameters. There are two dome shaped non-return valves with sockets for the breathing tubes in front; and a socket for the rebreathing bag behind. The control dials of the vaporisers are on the top of the assembly. There is no halothane vaporiser, but the ether vaporiser can be used for this purpose. The filler caps for the vaporisers are placed above the control dials. When the ether vaporiser contains halothane, a label or a piece of adhesive tape on the outside of the bottle should indicate its presence in writing.

Intermittent Flow Machines. Intermittent flow machines are designed to deliver nitrous oxide and oxygen intermittently on demand by the patient. The commonest British machine is the 'Walton Five' (Fig. 13). When the controls are opened mixed oxygen and nitrous oxide (in proportion to the setting on the control dial) fill a reservoir bag, flow ceasing automatically when full, until the patient inhales, when it fills again. The method is suitable for short operations in casualty departments and dental clinics. A Goldman Halothane vaporiser can be included in the circuit.

Entonox Apparatus. Designed originally for self administration of nitrous oxide and oxygen to induce analgesia during childbirth, the Entonox apparatus (page 177) is increasingly being used to alleviate pain and expand lung bases after upper abdominal and cardio-thoracic operations.

5 THE ANAESTHETIC ROOM—II

It is impossible to use an anaesthetic apparatus without some means of conveying oxygen, anaesthetic gases and vapours to the patient. The conventional Boyle's apparatus offers a choice of two methods. One known as the *Magill Attachment* is simple and the other which includes a means of absorbing expired carbon dioxide is rather more complicated.

MAGILL BREATHING ATTACHMENT*

The *Magill breathing attachment* was designed by Sir Ivan Magill more than fifty years ago to overcome the disadvantages of giving nitrous oxide, oxygen and ether from a large rebreathing bag held close to the patient's face which allowed free mixture of exhaled and fresh gases and resulted in undesirable accumulation of carbon dioxide. By removing the bag some distance from the patient, and putting an expiratory valve next to the facepiece exhaled gases pass out through the valve to the surrounding air, whilst fresh gases accumulate in the bag ready for the next inspiration. This modification also facilitated the development of endotracheal anaesthesia.

The Magill breathing attachment and British Standard com-

* *'British Standard' fittings.* In the past there has been lack of uniformity in the diameters of connections on anaesthetic apparatus made by different manufacturers (catheter mounts, angle pieces, and sockets for anaesthetic tubing) so that interchangeability was impossible. All new equipment manufactured in Great Britain or the U.S.A. must now conform to an agreed standard size so that all facepieces, endotracheal mounts, breathing hose mounts are interchangeable. All fittings have standard diameters from the gas outlets through to the face mask or endotracheal connection. The new standard uses a 'gender sequence'. Outlets are cone shaped ('male') to fit inside socket shaped ('female') inlets.

Several years may elapse before all apparatus conforms to the new standard. *Confusion can easily arise unless old and new parts are stored separately. Prior to use all parts should be connected from gas outlet to face mask or endotracheal mount to make sure there are no misfits.* The greatest difficulty will arise with endotracheal mounts. Older mounts are cone shaped and will not fit new cone shaped outlets.

ponents are shown in Fig. 14. Note that in the British Standard connection sequence the outlets are cone shaped and the inlets are socket shaped, i.e. gases flow from cones to sockets.

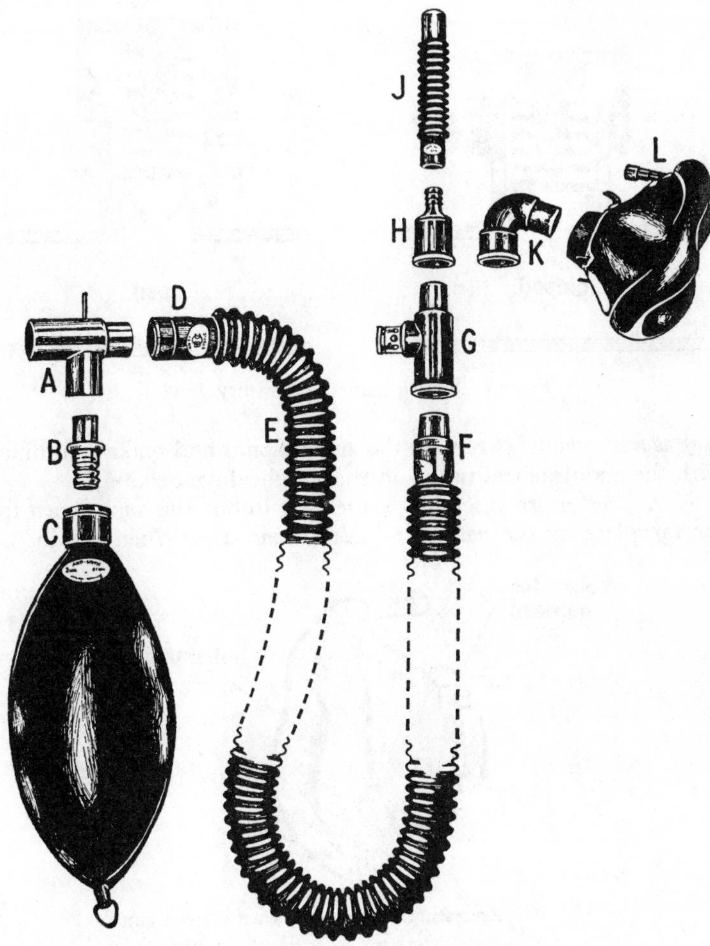

Fig. 14 Magill's breathing attachment
(*Note*. British Standard cone outlets and socket inlets)

A bag mount
B bag mount adaptor
C rebreathing bag
D adaptor
E corrugated tube
F adaptor, B.S. cone
G expiratory valve
H endotracheal adaptor
J adaptor tubing
K face mask angle mount
L face mask

For anaesthesia with a face mask, the *face mask angle mount* (K) connects the attachment to the *facepiece* (L).

For endotracheal anaesthesia (p. 59) an *endotracheal adaptor* (H)

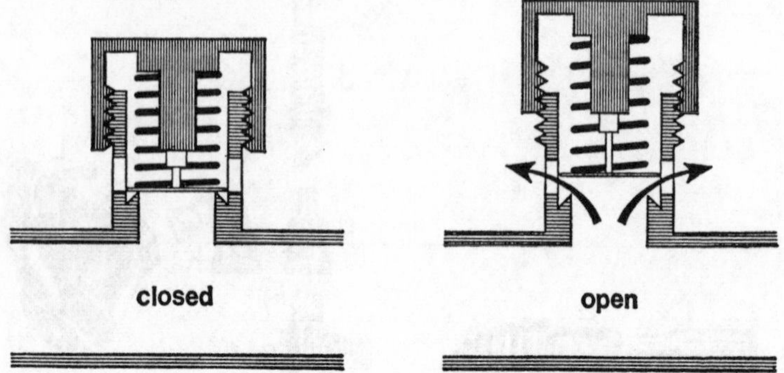

Fig. 15 Spring loaded expiratory valve

and *adaptor tubing* (J) replace the angle mount and make continuity with the endotracheal tube and endotracheal connection.

Note. The entire assembly is useless without the *angle mount* for the facepiece or the *endotracheal adaptor and tube.* When not in use

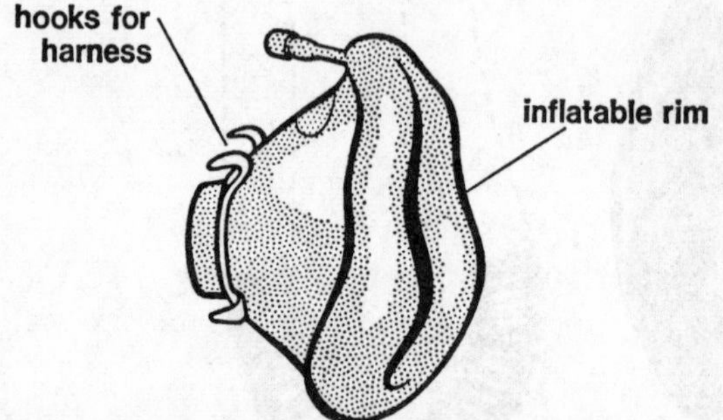

Fig. 16 Anaesthetic face mask with curved rim

these should always be kept on the anaesthetic machine. Two of each should be available in case one is mislaid.

The expiratory valve (Fig. 15) consists of a small metal plate covering a hole of similar size on the side of the straight metal mount. It is held in place by a covering metal screw cap and coiled spring. The screw controls the tension of the spring and thus the quantity of expired gases that pass out during expiration.

Face masks are of bakelite with antistatic rubber (p. 90), inflatable cushions, flat, or curved to the contours of the face to ensure a gas tight fit (Fig. 16). They are made in sizes suitable for infants, children and adults. A selection should be available before anaesthesia to allow choice of a size most suitable for the patient.

The facepiece harness. A facepiece harness is used to secure the mask to the patient's face during anaesthesia. There are 2 types:

Clausen's Harness (Fig. 17a) is a Y-shaped piece of rubber with perforations in the limbs of the Y which is placed behind the patient's head. The limbs of the Y are hooked on to a three hooked circular ring, which is slipped over the dome of the facepiece.

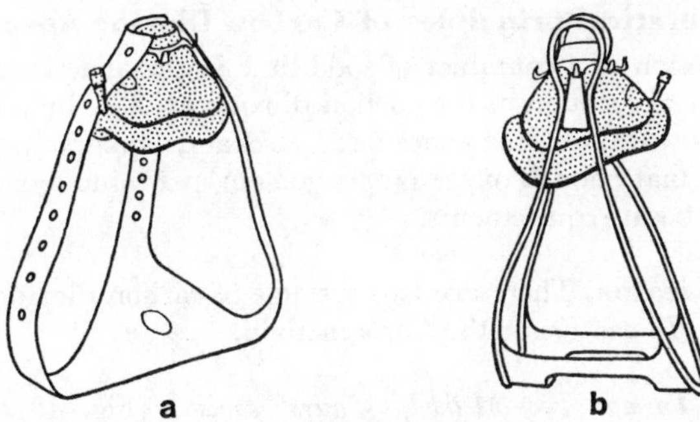

Fig. 17 Facepiece retaining harness

a Clausen b Connell

Connell's Harness (Fig. 17b) consists of a headpiece with pairs of rubber loops on either side. The loops slip through metal clips which allow easy adjustment and can be hooked on to studs on the side of the mask. Not all masks have these studs. Modern masks incorporate a five-pronged ring round the apex of the dome (Fig. 16) which permits the use of either pattern of harness.

A harness must always be available on the anaesthetic machine.

The Cardiff attachment. The Cardiff attachment allows the Magill breathing attachment to be placed at the right hand corner of the anaesthetic table instead of the back bracket. It consists of a movable metal socket to carry the breathing bag and is connected to the gas outlet at the top right hand end of the bracket carrying the flowmeters and vaporisers, so that manual compression of the rebreathing bag is possible without the need to stretch across the anaesthetic table.

CARBON DIOXIDE ABSORPTION APPARATUS

Carbon dioxide absorption and closed circuit. The Magill attachment is light and easy to handle, but the flow of gases must be at least seven litres per minute to prevent accumulation of carbon dioxide. This method is uneconomical when using expensive agents, and dangerous if the vapour is explosive, and was the reason for the introduction of carbon dioxide absorption techniques (familiar to Respiratory Physiologists for years) in 1937 when Dr Ralph Waters of Wisconsin introduced cyclopropane.

All modern machines should include an *Absorber Unit* because it allows the economical use of anaesthetic gases and of halothane.

Theoretical principles of Carbon Dioxide Absorption

The inclusion of a container of soda lime in the anaesthetic circuit allows the absorption of the carbon dioxide exhaled by the patient so that rebreathing of the anaesthetic gases and vapours is permissible provided that enough oxygen (250–300 cm^3 per minute) is added to meet the basal requirements.

Apparatus. There are two systems of carbon dioxide absorption. The *To and Fro* or the *Circle* method.

The To and Fro Method, Waters' canister (Fig. 18). Waters' canister consists of a cylindrical metal or plastic canister containing soda lime; a rebreathing bag; and a conical shaped mount incorporating an expiratory valve and side tube for fresh gases. An angle mount is provided for the face mask and an endotracheal adaptor and tube for endotracheal anaesthesia.

The canister must be placed as close to the patient as possible to ensure absorption of all the carbon dioxide, because gases in the space between the absorber and the patient are not cleared of carbon dioxide. Known as 'dead space' (p. 121), this should be kept as small as possible.

The method is cheap, simple, and can be used with any apparatus. Since the gases pass twice through the canister, it is an efficient method of carbon dioxide absorption but it is difficult to secure the heavy canister close to the patient's face during certain operations, although fixing devices are available.

Circle Absorption Systems. Circle absorption systems were designed to overcome the disadvantage of an absorber close to the face by attaching it to the anaesthetic trolley, gases being carried by separate corrugated breathing tubes to and from the absorber

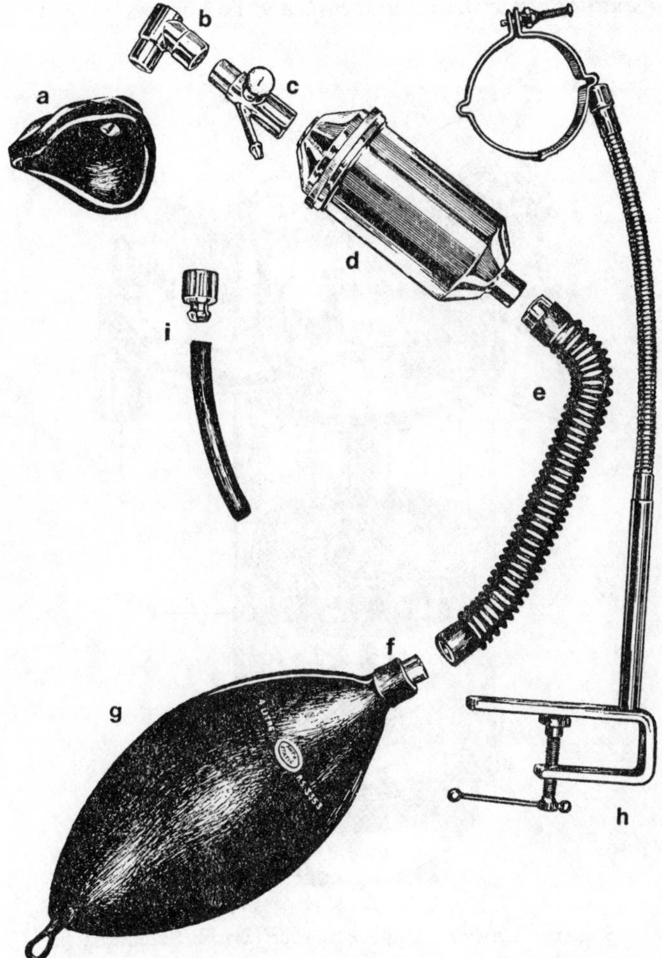

Fig. 18 Waters' canister and attachments

a face mask
b angle piece
c expiratory valve mount with gas feed
d Waters' canister
e corrugated extension tubing and mounts
f bag mount
g rebreathing bag
h flexible support for canister
i endotracheal mount and tubing

which contains unidirectional 'non-return' valves so that inspiratory and expiratory gases travel in a *circle* and do not mix.

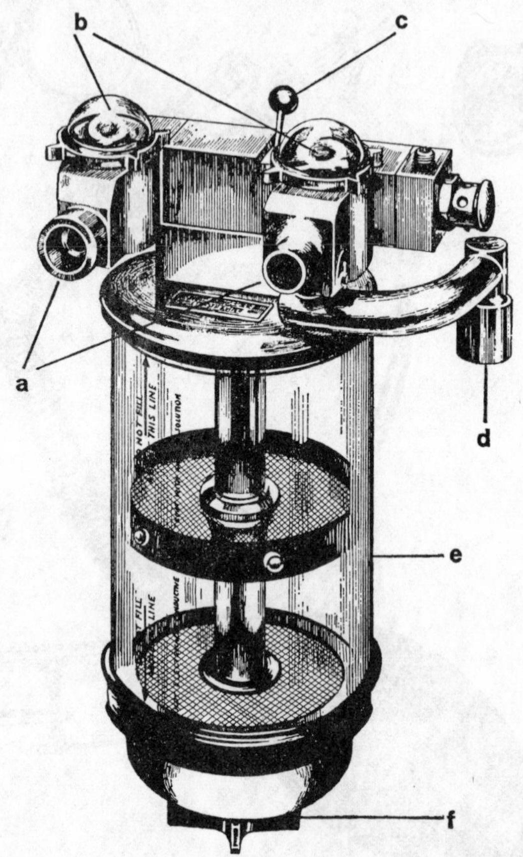

Fig. 19 Carbon dioxide absorber (British Standard)

a socket inlet and cone outlet ports
b 'non-return' valves
c 'on-off' control
d mount for reservoir bag
e soda lime canister
f release screw

Several types of apparatus are manufactured. Although differing in appearance all have the following in common (Fig. 19):

(i) A container for soda lime (transparent in modern models).
(ii) 'Inlet' and 'outlet' ports with unidirectional valves for expiratory and inspiratory tubing.
(iii) A reservoir bag.

(iv) An ON/OFF control to allow gases to by-pass the soda lime when required (e.g. to change the soda lime).

(v) An inlet for fresh gases.

Figure 20 shows the breathing attachments for a circle absorption system. Separate breathing tubes (a and b) are connected proximally

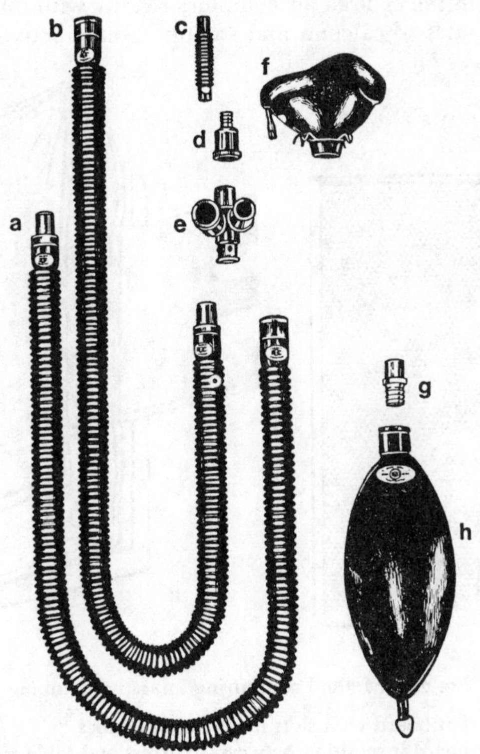

Fig. 20 Breathing attachment for circle absorber (British Standard)

a expiratory tubing
b inspiratory tubing
c endotracheal adaptor tubing
d endotracheal adaptor
e Y-piece and expiratory valve
f face mask
g bag mount
h rebreathing bag

to the absorber unit and distally to the Y-piece a metal swivel mount and expiratory valve (e) for the face mask or endotracheal connector and tubing (c and d).

The assembly is rather heavy and unless supported will tend to displace the face mask or endotracheal tube. The absorber should be raised to the level of the patient and the tubing clipped to the pillow or fixed into clefts on a piece of flat board (Fig. 21) which is kept for this purpose under the mattress of the operating table.

Soda Lime. Soda lime is a mixture of 90% calcium hydroxide (quick lime) and 5% sodium hydroxide (caustic soda) with silicates added to prevent powder formation. Carbon dioxide, in the presence of moisture in the expired air combines readily with this mixture to form carbonates of calcium and sodium. Anaesthetic soda lime is

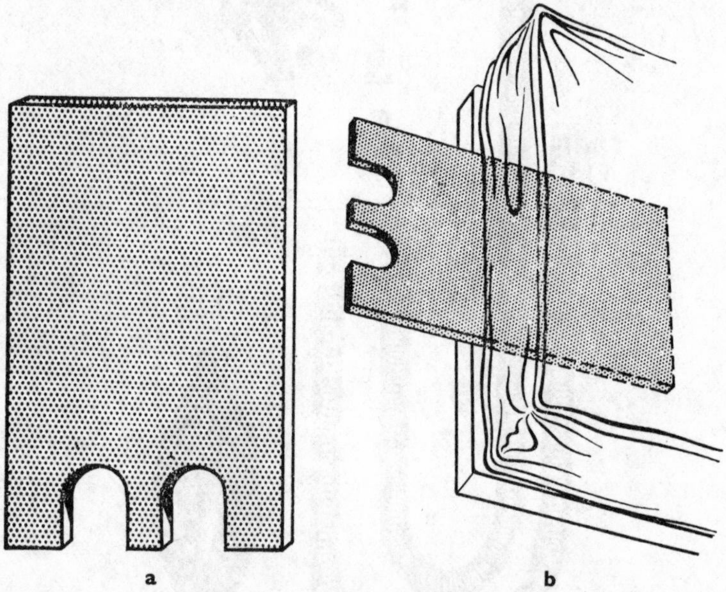

Fig. 21 Method of securing anaesthetic tubing

a flat board with slots for breathing tubes
b board in position between mattress and table top

made in granules of uniform size to ensure maximum efficiency of absorption and minimum resistance to respiration. Soda lime becomes exhausted when the alkaline sodium and calcium hydroxides are saturated with carbonic acid gas. Chemical indicators are added to soda lime, which change colour when it becomes exhausted. 'Durasorb' changes from *pink* to *white*; 'Calona' from *cream* to *violet*; and 'Sofnol' from *green* to *brown*.

A one-pound canister of soda lime becomes exhausted after *3–4 hours* of *continuous use* but some regeneration of activity occurs if the soda lime is rested for two hours, allowing up to *six hours* of *intermittent use*.

Changing Soda Lime

Waters' Canister. A duplicate canister should be available to replace the exhausted one when required. The used canister can then be opened by unscrewing and its contents replaced by fresh granules. Care should be taken to screw the canister firmly so that there is no 'play', otherwise a leak will occur when next used. If the canister is not transparent, the date and time of changing should be indicated by a strip of adhesive tape.

Circle Absorbers. Large canisters on newer circle absorbers hold two pounds of soda lime which will remain active for periods of up to 6 hours continuous use or 12 hours intermittent use. The canister is easily removed by loosening a handscrew at its underside. Unless the screw is fully tightened when replacing the canister the circuit will leak. In some models this has been overcome by fitting a quick action release device.

SUCTION EQUIPMENT

Suction may be required at any time and apparatus should be available for the sole use of the anaesthetist, apart from that provided for the surgeon. It can be supplied in one of three forms: piped, mechanical, or by the jet principle.

Piped suction. In suites with centrally installed suction an outlet is placed alongside those for anaesthetic gases. A suction bottle is connected to it by pressure tubing.

Mechanical suction apparatus. Suction is provided by an electric motor which drives a small suction pump. Some models have one bottle and on others there are two, with a switch to transfer suction to the second bottle when the first one is full.

'Jet' type suction. This method utilises the 'Venturi' or jet principle whereby compressed air, steam, or water is driven under pressure through a jet which sucks in air through an opening just beyond it in the side of the tube. This method of suction is incorporated in some anaesthetic machines, the jet being provided from an oxygen cylinder and regulated by a foot pedal or hand operated screw.

Suction Ends, Connections and Catheters

Suction Ends are used during and after operation to remove fluid, blood, mucus, etc. from the mouth and pharynx. They consist of a metal or plastic handle and tubing, bent to pass over the tongue into the pharynx. A 'universal' handle allows use of different suction

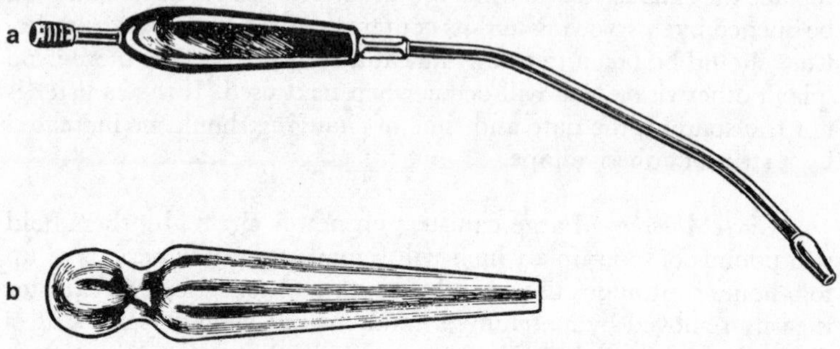

Fig. 22 Suction ends

a Yankauer b Frenchay Hospital perspex

ends. The *Yankauer suction end* (Fig. 22a) of plastic or metal is a useful general purpose instrument. The *Frenchay perspex suction end* (Fig. 22b) is shorter than other suction ends and serves equally well as a *suction connection.*

Suction connections connect suction tubing to *suction catheters.* They should be transparent in order to reveal the nature and

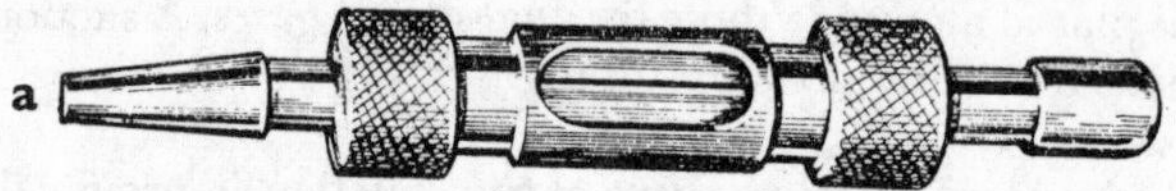

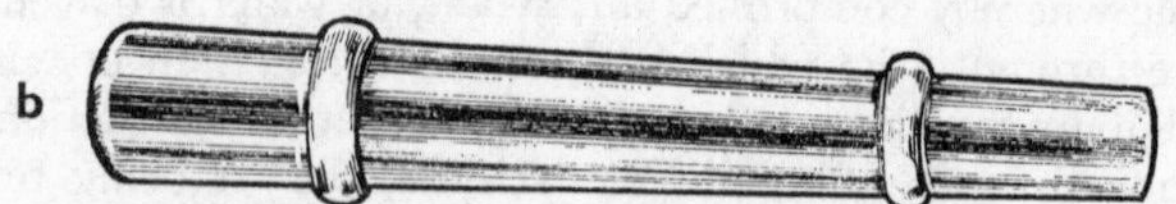

Fig. 23 Suction connections

a Corney visual b Frenchay Hospital perspex

quantity of fluid removed. There are two common patterns: The *Corney visual suction connection* (Fig. 23a) is metal with tapered ends and a transparent window. It is unbreakable, and can be dismantled for sterilisation. The *Frenchay perspex suction connection* (Fig. 23b) is about 7·5 cm long with one end for a catheter and the other, slightly broader, for the suction tubing.

Note. Glass suction connections should never be used because they break too easily.

Suction Catheters. Endobronchial suction catheters are intended for removal of secretions from the trachea and bronchi, during or after anaesthetics. A supply of sterile catheters should be kept ready with the suction apparatus. They may be either disposable or of rubber, or gum elastic which need cleaning and re-sterilising after use.

AIRWAYS

Airways are curved tubes of metal or rubber, which on insertion into the mouth slide over the tongue with their end resting in the

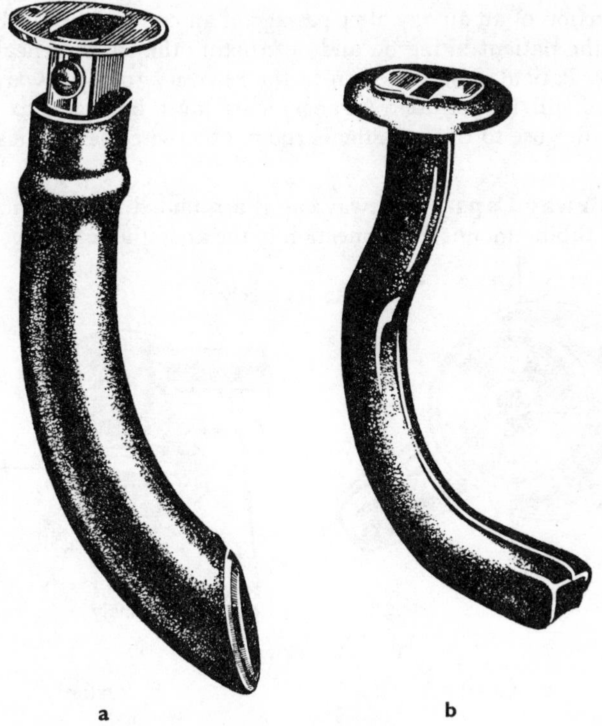

Fig. 24 Airways

a Phillips pattern b Guedel pattern

c

pharynx, thus preventing the tongue falling back and obstructing respiration, and are used to keep a clear airway during anaesthesia and recovery (Fig. 24). There are several types:

The *Phillips Airway*: is of rounded *rubber* with a metal mount *flattened* in cross section.

Hewitt's Airway: is similar to the Phillips but has a *circular* metal mount.

Hirsch Airway: is also similar to Phillips, but has a side tube on the metal mount for rubber tubing carrying oxygen and/or anaesthetic vapour.

Guedel Airway: more exactly shaped to the tongue, made of black, white or transparent rubber with a metal plated insert to give extra rigidity between the teeth.

Waters' Airway: is the same shape as the Guedel, but made entirely of metal and available with or without a side tube.

All airways are available in four sizes, *size 1* (for infants) being the *smallest*, and *size 4 the largest*. A supply of sterilised airways should be kept on the anaesthetic trolley.

Insertion of an airway after passage of an endotracheal tube prevents the patient biting on and obstructing the endotracheal tube.

Note. Patients always return to the recovery room or ward with airways still in position. Arrangements must be made to return them after use to the anaesthetic room, otherwise they are lost.

Airway Caps. An airway cap is a rounded metal attachment with a tubing mount for connection to the anaesthetic tubing, which

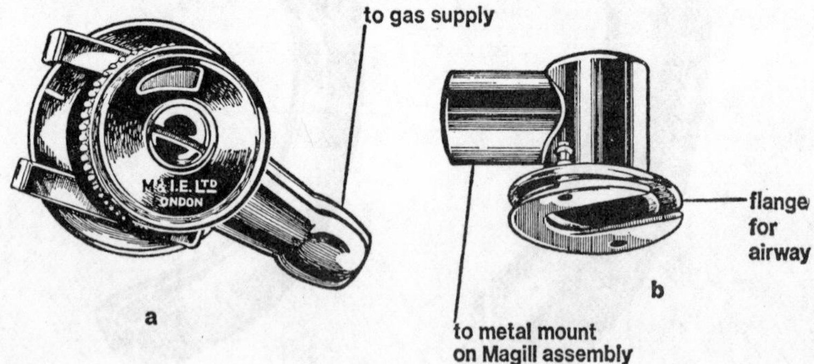

Fig. 25 Airway caps

a Charles b Oxford

can be attached to the metal flange of a Phillips or Guedel airway to maintain anaesthesia when a face mask would interfere with the surgeon, but where for technical reasons passage of an endotracheal tube is not desired (e.g. in ophthalmic surgery). There are two

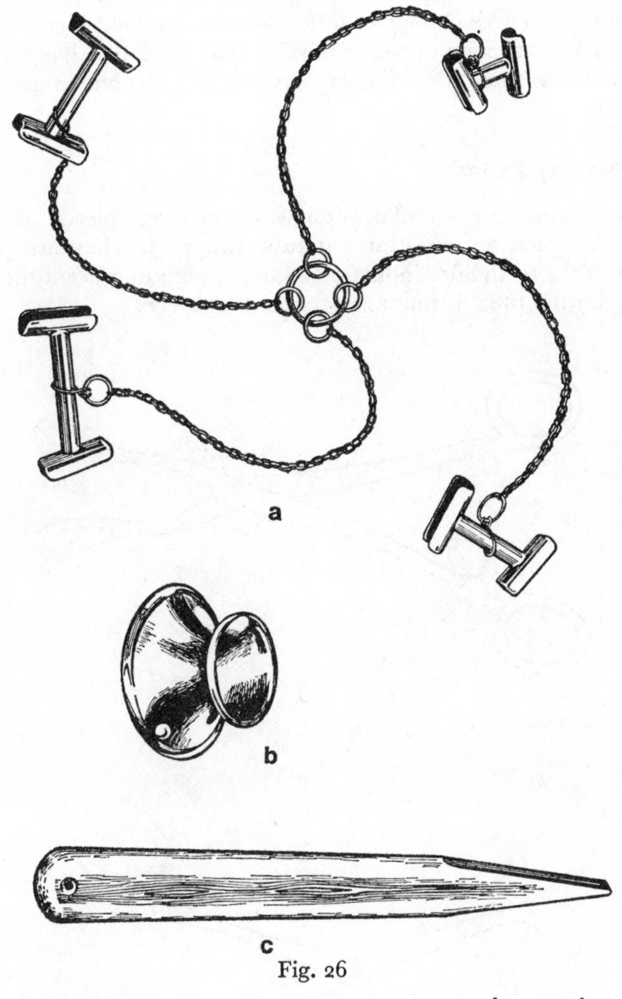

Fig. 26

a mouth props b airway prop c wooden mouth wedge

types: (i) the *Charles airway cap* (Fig. 25a) has a round mobile side tube for connection to the gas supply by rubber tubing or a tubing mount. (ii) The *Oxford airway cap* (Fig. 25b) has a side tube which joins the gas supply through the expiratory valve mount.

Mouth Props

Mouth props are small, rounded or rectangular pieces of metal, rubber, or plastic designed to 'prop' open the mouth during dental anaesthesia. Three or four of different sizes are held together by a chain. After selection of one of suitable size, the others hang outside the mouth so there is no danger of swallowing the one in use.

Airway Props

Airway props are circular, hollow or grooved pieces of metal through which an endotracheal tube can pass. They are placed between the teeth after induction of anaesthesia to prevent the teeth biting on the tube during anaesthesia or recovery.

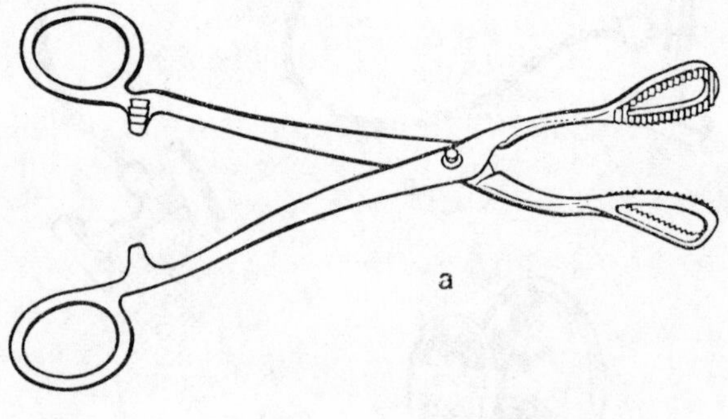

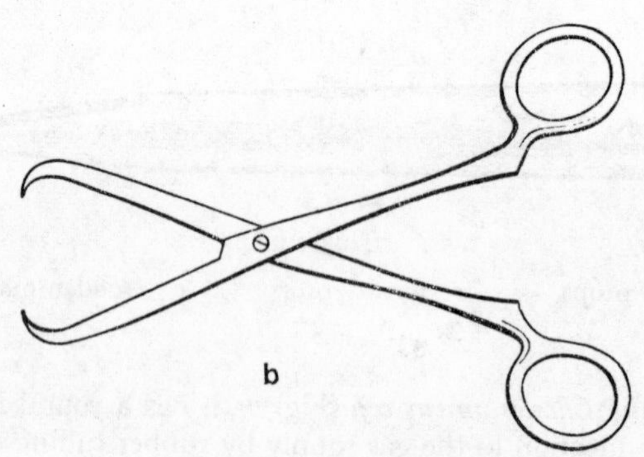

Fig. 27 Tongue forceps
a Guy's b Moynihan

The Mouth Wedge

The mouth wedge (Hewitt's) is a rounded piece of boxwood about 10 cm long and of 13 mm diameter, wedge-shaped at one end. It is used to open clenched jaws by pressing the wedge gently but firmly between the incisor teeth. It may be needed during recovery to relieve obstruction of respiration.

Tongue Forceps

Tongue forceps are used to grasp the tongue and pull it forward to clear the airway after operations on the tongue or the back of the throat where insertion of an airway may not be practicable. There are two common varieties: (i) *Guy's Pattern* (Fig. 27a) The ends are flat and serrated to grasp the tongue by compression, which, unless done gently can produce extensive bruising. (ii) *Moynihan's tongue forceps* (Fig. 27b). The ends are sharp. Though savage in appearance, this pattern is less traumatic than Guy's.

MOUTH GAGS

Mouth gags serve two purposes: (i) *to keep open an already relaxed jaw* (as, for example, during dental surgery or operations on the tongue

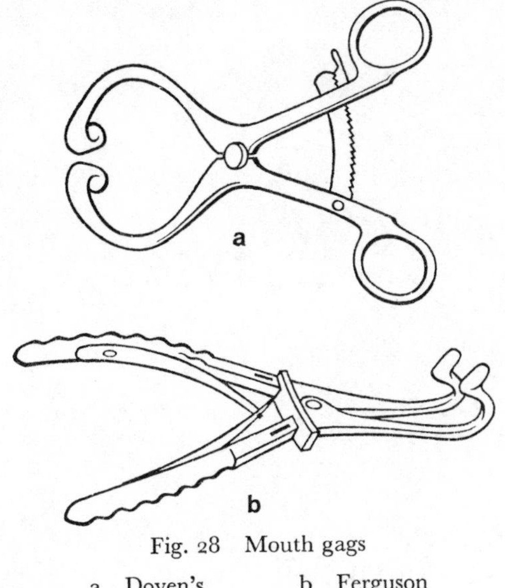

Fig. 28 Mouth gags

a Doyen's b Ferguson

or cheek) or (ii) *to force open a clenched jaw* (prior to insertion of an airway, suction, or application of tongue forceps).

(i) *Gags for fixing open a relaxed jaw* are associated with the name of *Doyen* (Fig. 28a) and have semi-circular blades curved on the flat to lie close to the cheek. The 'bite' is grooved and lined with lead to prevent slipping, when inserted between the teeth. The shape of the 'bite' makes it obvious that it could not be inserted between clenched teeth. A ratchet locking device keeps the gag open.

(ii) *Gags for insertion between clenched teeth are associated* with the name of *Ferguson*, *Mason* and *Ackland* (Fig. 28b). All have thin blades for insertion between the back (molar) teeth. (To attempt to force open by pressure on the front teeth would be most hazardous.) The blades of the Mason gag are in apposition when closed, but those of the Ferguson-Ackland modification lie in the same plane and thus are just that little bit more narrow. It is unnecessary to cover the blades with rubber because it increases difficulty of insertion between clenched teeth. A sliding ratchet on the handles operated by the thumb and forefinger keeps the blades apart when opened.

6 THE ANAESTHETIC ROOM—III

EQUIPMENT FOR ENDOTRACHEAL INTUBATION ANAESTHESIA

Endotracheal intubation is the passage of a curved (rubber) tube into the trachea, through the nose (*nasal intubation*) or through the mouth (*oral intubation*) (Fig. 29). The nasal route is used for operations on the mouth and tongue, including extraction of teeth. Apparatus for intubation consists of (1) a Laryngoscope. (2) Endotracheal tubes. (3) Magill's endotracheal introducing forceps. (4) Endotracheal mounts and connections. (5) Local anaesthetic spray. (6) Catheter lubricant; throat packs; adhesive tape; a 20 ml syringe to inflate cuffed tubes, and a clip to close the end of the inflating tube.

(1) Laryngoscopes. Laryngoscopes were originally designed by ear, nose and throat surgeons to examine the *interior* of the larynx as well as the vocal cords. Anaesthetic laryngoscopes are designed only to bring the vocal cords into view so that a tube can be passed through them into the larynx without obstruction from the tongue. An anaesthetic laryngoscope consists of a *handle* and a *flat blade* carrying a light bulb. The handle is cylindrical and contains two 1·5 volt batteries. Its upper end is slotted to take the blade which is secured by a clip or screw, but which can move through a right angle, being alongside the handle when not in use and at right angles to it when ready for use. On extension, contacts in the handle and blade approximate so that the bulb in the blade is illuminated by the batteries in the handle.

Laryngoscope blades are straight (Magill pattern) or *curved* (Mackintosh pattern) and each is available in four sizes: large, medium, small (for children), and very small (for infants). All will fit the same handle. The *straight* (*Magill*) *blade* exposes the vocal cords when passed over the tongue into the pharynx so that its tip comes to rest in *front* of the epiglottis, which is then lifted *forwards* by a backward movement of the handle (Fig. 30) to reveal the laryngeal aperture. The *curved* (Mackintosh) blade is introduced in the same way, but its tip comes to rest in the groove *between* the epiglottis and the base of the tongue (i.e. *behind* the epiglottis). A similar forward movement of the tip by a backward movement of the handle brings the vocal cords into view.

Laryngoscopes should always be tested before use by extending the blade on the handle to its fullest extent to make certain the light

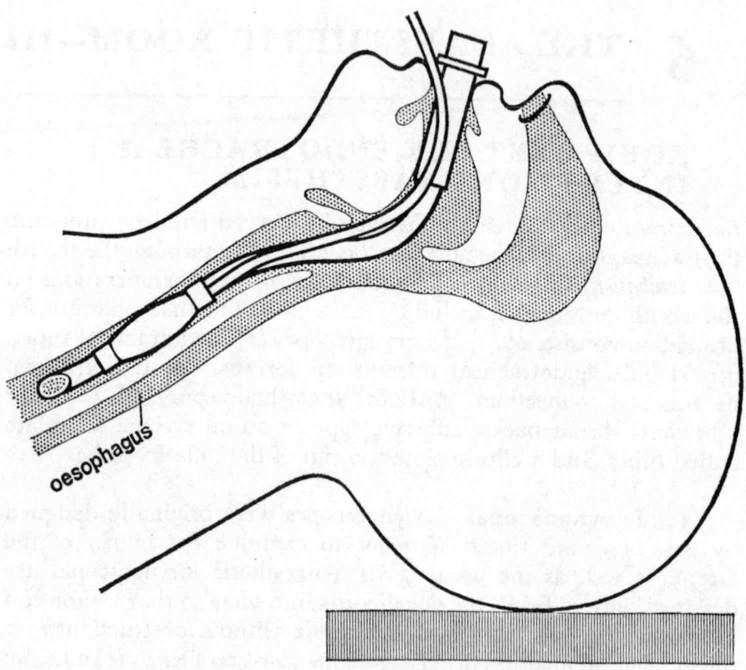

Fig. 29 Endotracheal tube in position

shines brightly. If the light is dim or intermittent, it should be withdrawn from use until the fault has been corrected. Some commoner causes of failure are:

(i) The bulb may be loose and need tightening. It lies in a slot half way along the blade and should be screwed home securely.

(ii) If tightening fails to produce a light, the bulb should be changed. A number of new bulbs should be kept in a small box, clearly labelled.

(iii) If the batteries have not been changed recently, they may need replacing. This is done by unscrewing the cap at the base of the handle.

(iv) Failure of all the above measures suggests that the contacts must be faulty. Sometimes they become covered with lubricant. If cleaning with spirit fails to produce a light, the instrument should be sent for repair.

Note. Two laryngoscopes should always be available. In spite of a satisfactory test before use the light may fail just at the moment of exposure of the larynx. Lack of a spare instrument invites disaster.

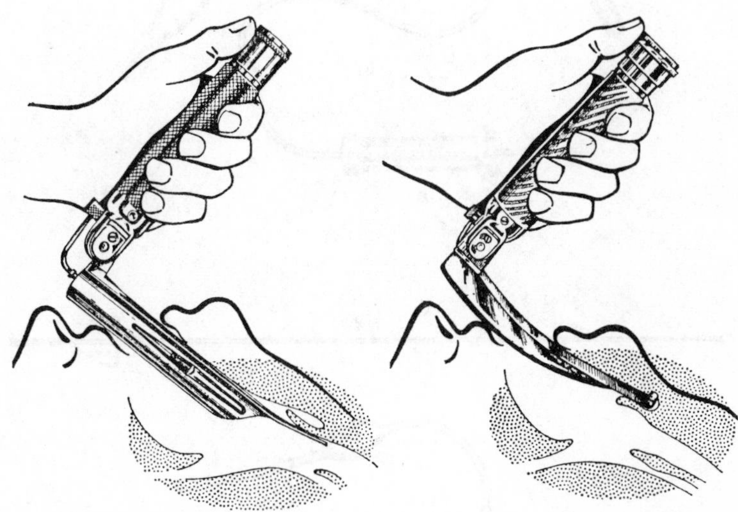

Magill laryngoscope in position MacIntosh laryngoscope in position

Fig. 30

(2) Endotracheal Tubes. The standard endotracheal tubes are widely known as Magill's tubes (after the anaesthetist Sir Ivan Magill, who designed them). They are tubes of rubber or plastic, 38 centimetres in length, curved in a half circle with one end bevelled to facilitate insertion through the larynx. There are eleven sizes, 0 to 10 according to the internal diameter which varies from 3 to 9 mm.

There are two types—*plain* (or 'uncuffed') and *cuffed. Plain tubes* may be passed through the mouth, or through the nose if the presence of a tube in the mouth could interfere with the operation: for example on the tongue, the jaws, or during dental extractions. When the nasal route is used a sponge or paraffin-soaked pack should be available to place in the back of the throat to prevent seepage of blood or mucus around the tube into the trachea. (The operation of tonsillectomy is an exception. Here, the head being extended, blood accumulates in the back of the pharynx from whence it can be removed by suction.)

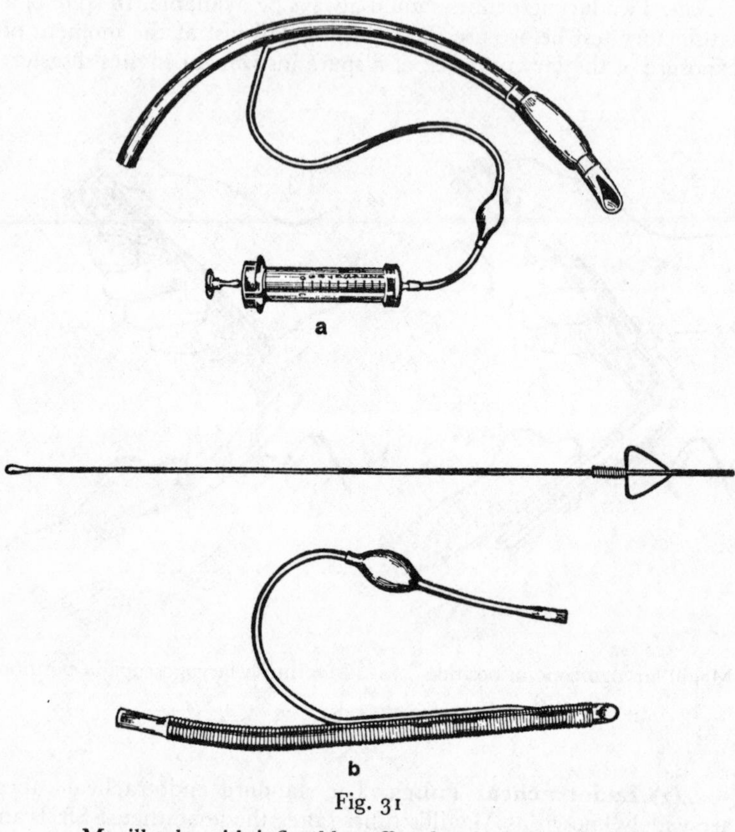

Fig. 31

a Magill tube with inflatable cuff and syringe for inflating cuff
b nylon reinforced tube with introducer

Cuffed tubes have an inflatable rubber cuff with inflating tube and 'pilot balloon'. The cuff is vulcanised on the outer side of the tube about 12 mm from its end. After insertion of the tube the cuff is inflated with air to provide an airtight seal round the trachea, thus preventing reflux of gases round the tube during inflation of the lungs, or seepage of blood or secretions into the trachea (Fig. 31a).

Choice of size and length of tubes. The smallest sizes, 0–2 are suitable for infants; sizes 3–5 for young children; 5–7 for teenagers and 8–10 for adults.

New tubes should be cut to a convenient length before use. Nasal tubes should approximate to the distance between the lobe of the ear and the tip of the nose, for passage through the mouth they should be eight centimetres shorter.

Testing Tubes before Use

All except new tubes should be tested for weaknesses before use because sterilisation by heat softens the rubber of walls and cuffs.

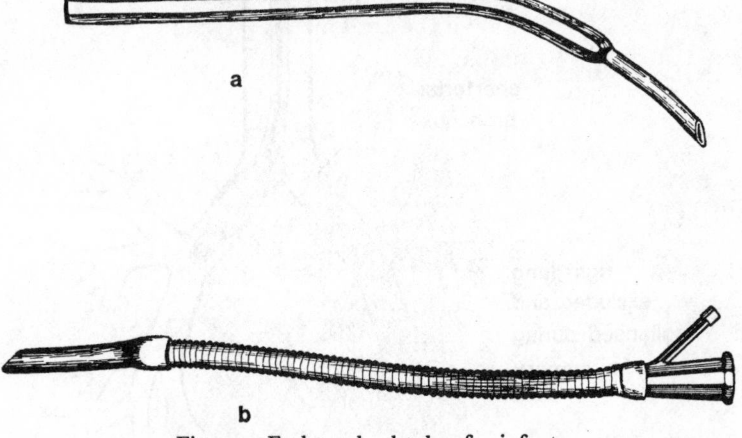

Fig. 32 Endotracheal tubes for infants

a Cole's or Riplex tube
b Magill's flexometallic tube with metal mount and side tube

Softening of the wall can be detected by bending the tubes until the ends approximate when a soft tube will kink. Softening of the cuff is evident from ballooning of part of the wall in inflation. (Failure to inflate of course indicates rupture of the cuff.)

Tubes which show these deficiencies should be discarded because kinking of the tube or ballooning of the cuff are both possible causes of obstructed respiration during anaesthesia.

Special Endotracheal Tubes

Apart from the standard endotracheal tubes there are others designed for uses on special occasions. These are (i) nylon reinforced tubes, (ii) tubes for infants, and (iii) endobronchial tubes for use in open chest operations.

(i) *Nylon reinforced flexible tubes* are made of latex rubber with a stout coil of nylon embedded in their walls (Fig. 31b). Normally they are straight, but possess the useful property of bending in any direction without kinking. They are intended for use in circumstances where flexion of the head after intubation might cause kinking of a soft rubber tube. They should always be available for neurosurgical procedures or when the operation involves turning the patient on the face ('prone' position). 'Cuffed' and 'plain' tubes are

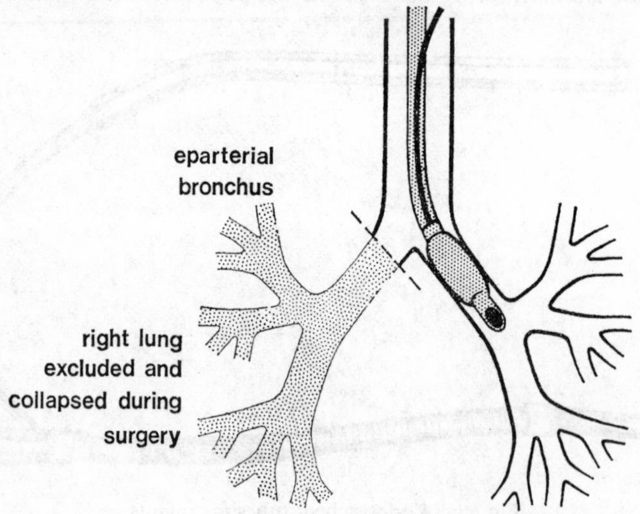

Fig. 33 Left endobronchial tube to allow anaesthesia through left lung during surgery on right lung

available. In some the cuff is detachable and can be changed when necessary because these tubes do not soften or deteriorate after repeated sterilisation as quickly as rubber cuffs.

A malleable copper wire introducer (Fig. 31) is essential for passage of flexible tubes and should be well lubricated before use.

(ii) *Infants' endotracheal tubes*. Although the standard Magill endotracheal tubes include those small enough for infants there are also tubes embodying special features for paediatric use. These are: (*a*) *The Cole or Riplex tubes* (Fig. 32a). The terminal 3 centimetres of the tube are small enough to pass through the infantile larynx, but the remainder is of a larger diameter to reduce resistance to respiration. (*b*) *Magill flexometallic tube* (Fig. 32b). A coil of stainless steel wire or stout nylon is incorporated into the latex wall of the tube, except for the terminal 3 centimetres, which are of rubber. A trumpet-shaped metal mount with a gas feed inlet attached to the open end, which functions as a modified Ayre's 'T' piece (page 71). It can be used with any apparatus which can provide a supply of oxygen and anaesthetic vapour. Rhythmic inflation of the lungs can be performed by simply placing a finger over the metal end and releasing it at regular intervals.

(iii) *Endobronchial tubes for use during operations through the chest.* Several tubes have been designed to allow maintenance of anaesthesia in one lung, whilst blocking off the lung on the side of the chest undergoing operation, allowing it to collapse to give the surgeon a clear operative field. A long tube with a short cuff will pass naturally into the *left main bronchus* and after inflation of the cuff, the right lung is isolated so that it collapses (Fig. 33). Passage into the *right lung* is more difficult because the right bronchus is at a sharper angle than the left, whilst the presence of the eparterial bronchus (Fig. 33), a short distance from the carina makes it difficult to place a cuffed tube without occluding this and collapsing the right upper lobe as well as the left lung. Several tubes have been designed to overcome this and other problems. Their description would take too much space and the interested reader is referred to the catalogues of Anaesthetic Equipment Manufacturers where these tubes are well described and illustrated.

Lubricants. Lubricants—*water soluble* (jelly) or *oily* (smeared vaseline) on the outside of the endotracheal tube ease their passage and reduce the likelihood of damage to the larynx and trachea. Some contain a local analgesic to reduce reflex coughing initiated by contact of tube and tracheal mucous membrane. Water soluble lubricants are preferable to those containing vaseline which causes rapid deterioration and softening of rubber tubes.

(3) Magill's endotracheal introducing forceps (Fig. 34). Magill's introducing forceps are designed to grasp the end of the endotracheal tube in the back of the throat and direct it gently into the laryngeal aperture during *nasal intubation.* It has a 'dinner fork' curve on the flat which enables the anaesthetist to reach over the back of the tongue into the pharynx.

(4) The endotracheal adaptor mount* and tube (Fig. 35) consists of an adaptor tube—a short length of corrugated rubber or nylon reinforced tubing about 13 millimetres in diameter, which is

* Endotracheal adaptors are also known as *Catheter Mounts.* The term dates back to the days when gum-elastic catheters were passed into the trachea, and anaesthesia maintained by blowing ether vapour into the lungs.

attached to a hard rubber endotracheal adaptor, socket shaped to fit into the cone shaped outlet of the anaesthetic hose.

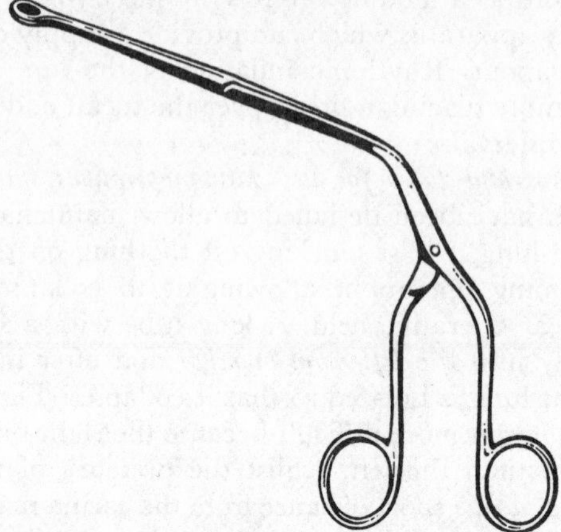

Fig. 34 Magill's introducing forceps

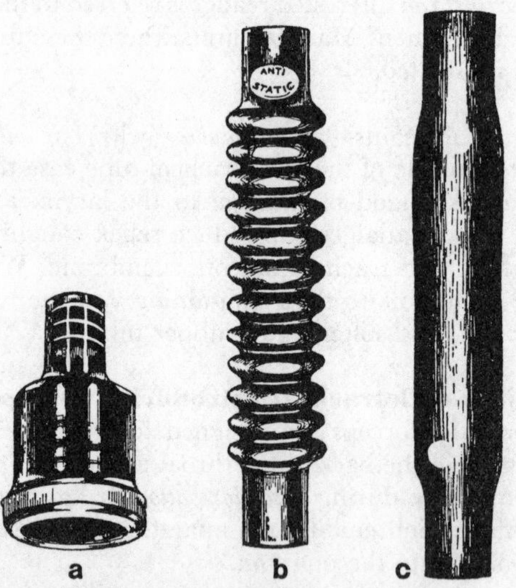

Fig. 35 Endotracheal adaptors and adaptor tubes
a anti-static, hard rubber adaptor b corrugated adaptor tube
c nylon reinforced adaptor tube

There should be two endotracheal mounts on each machine, because should one become mislaid it is impossible to continue the anaesthetic.

Endotracheal Connections

Endotracheal connections are curved metal tubes which join the endotracheal tube to the adaptor mount, each known by the name

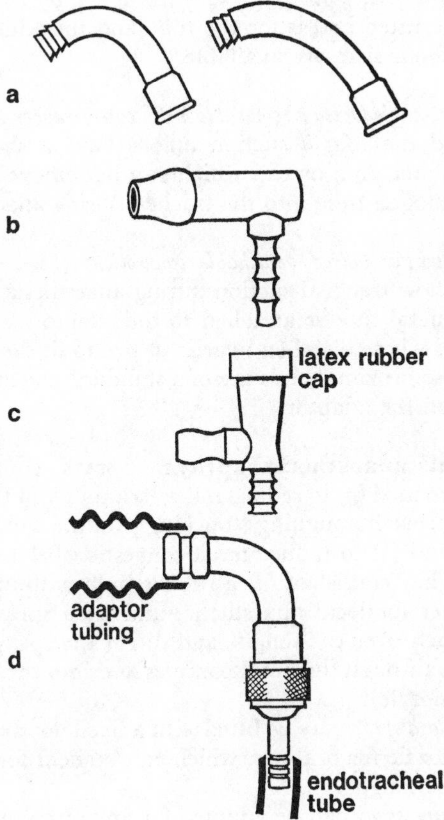

Fig. 36 Endotracheal connections

a curved (Magill)
b right-angled plain (Rowbotham)
c right-angled with removable cap
d paired detachable (Nosworthy)

of the anaesthetist who designed it. For descriptive purposes there are four main designs: (i) *Curved*; (ii) *Right-angled*; (iii) *Right-angled with removable cap*; (iv) *Paired detachable.*

(i) *Curved connections.* These are known as *Magill* connections (Fig. 36a). One end is serrated for the endotracheal tube and the other expanded for the tube mount (Fig. 36a). There are 16 different sizes. Some, having a sharp curve, are intended to use with nasal tubes and others, longer and more gently curved, are for oral tubes.

(ii) *Right-angled, plain* (Fig. 36b). Designed by *Dr S. Rowbotham*, the tapered serrated end is for the tube and the wider end for the tube mount. Four sizes are available.

(iii) *Right-angled with a removable metal cap or rubber plug* (Fig. 36c). The *Cobb* and the *Magill* suction unions have a short projection carrying a rubber plug or cap which can be removed to allow the passage of a suction tube into the trachea during anaesthesia.

(iv) *Nosworthy paired detachable connections* (Fig. 36d) are also designed to allow tracheal suction during anaesthesia.

A curved metal tube is attached to the adaptor. There are four separate tubes whose distal end varies in size to fit the endotracheal tube but whose proximal ends are of a standard size and fit into the curved tube on the adaptor.

(5) Local anaesthetic sprays. Sprays containing local anaesthetic are used (*a*) to reduce reflex irritability of the larynx and trachea and prevent coughing ('bucking') on the tube during light anaesthesia, and (*b*) to reduce nasal congestion before passage of a nasal tube. They consist of (*a*) a rubber bulb with air valve, (*b*) a small container for local anaesthetic, and (*c*) a spray nozzle long enough to reach over the tongue and direct the spray through the larynx or pass through the nasal passages and into the pharynx (e.g. Rowbotham nozzle).

The Mackintosh spray may be fitted with a fixed nozzle for nasal use, or a pliable nozzle for oral use, which can be bent for passing over the back of the tongue.

The Multicaine spray can be adapted for any purpose by attaching different nozzles, all of which are interchangeable.

Solutions in common use are: *Cocaine*, in strength varying from 4% to 20%; Lignocaine 4%, and Amethocaine 1%. All are poisonous if given in excess. Cocaine must be kept in the D.D.A. cupboard and only taken out when the anaesthetist wishes to refill the nebuliser.

The Emergency Bronchoscope. A bronchoscope is a long, thin, slightly oval metal tube about 46 cm in length, small enough to pass through the larynx, down the trachea and into the left or right main bronchus. It carries a light towards its further end which, in types used for special examinations, connects to a battery or transformer. It is used (*a*) to pass endobronchial tubes, and (*b*) to remove secretions or inhaled vomitus from trachea and bronchi. For this last procedure it will be required urgently so one is always kept in readiness in an easily accessible place and is known as the *Emergency Bronchoscope*.

To be ready at short notice and used anywhere it is fitted with a *detachable handle* like the laryngoscope to allow a quick change of blade. The Magill emergency bronchoscope has four blades, the largest having an internal diameter of 11 mm, the next 8 mm, then 5 mm, and 3 mm. The last two are suitable for children and infants. At the proximal end of the bronchoscope there is a short side tube for attachment to a source of oxygen or to the anaesthetic machine by means of a length of rubber tubing.

The emergency bronchoscope should be kept in an accessible place, clearly marked in a box. As it is not frequently required, it should be regularly examined to ensure that it is in working order. A 'non-leak' battery should be used.

MODIFIED EQUIPMENT FOR INFANTS AND SMALL CHILDREN

Anaesthesia for infants and small children presents special problems because the amount of air they breathe, and the size of their air passages are relatively much smaller than an adult or a child of 7 or 8 years of age. So little is air taken in at each breath that rebreathing with conventional circuits results in accumulation of excessive amounts of carbon dioxide. The diameter of the trachea in relation to the size of the lungs being less than in older subjects, the presence of an endotracheal tube greatly increases *resistance to breathing*. During paediatric anaesthesia rebreathing is avoided and resistance to breathing kept as small as possible by the use of (i) the 'open' method, (ii) non-return valves, (iii) the Ayre's 'T' piece, (iv) endotracheal tubes of special design. 'Paediatric sets' are available which embody some or all of these devices.

(i) The Open Method. The open method is the oldest way of inducing and maintaining anaesthesia but is seldom used except for infants and children. Liquid anaesthetic is dropped from a 'drop' bottle on to a piece of lint or gauze stretched over a wire mask and held over the patient's face. A 'drop' bottle is a medicine bottle with a cork through which two fine hollow tubes pass. On holding the bottle head downwards, the anaesthetic drops through one tube whilst air passes down into the bottle through the other to replace the liquid which has emerged. The wire mask is known as the 'Schimmelbusch' mask. A square piece of 'gamgee' tissue covers the face, to protect the eyes and provides an airtight seal between the mask and the face.

(ii) Non-return valves are designed to eliminate rebreathing entirely. They are attached to the face-piece or endotracheal mount.

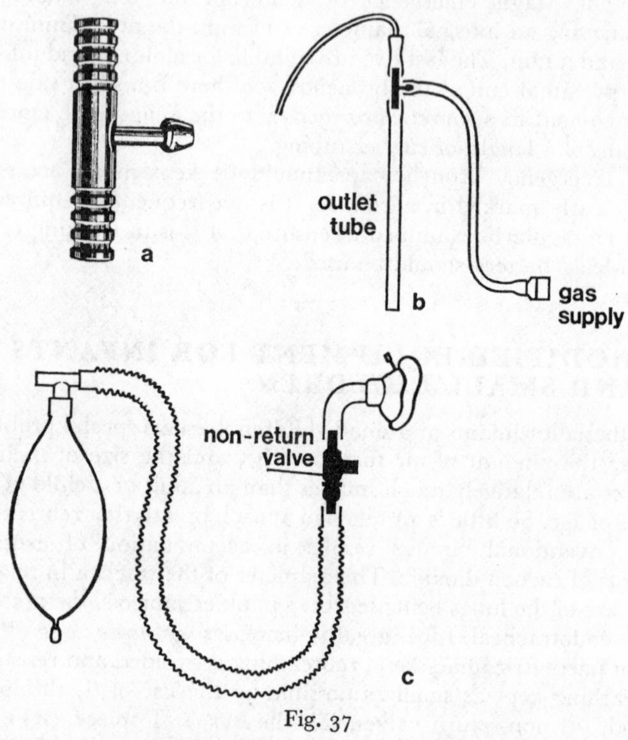

Fig. 37

a Ayre's 'T' piece
b method of using Ayre's 'T' piece
c method of using 'non-return' valves

On expiration a valve closes diverting gases to the outside air. The valve must be light and move easily in order to keep resistance to respiration as low as possible. There are three types in use:

(*a*) *The Ruben Valve*. A light rather fragile transparent piece of equipment. The non-return valve can be seen to slide back and forth during respiration. The *red* mount is for connection to the patient and the *blue* to the gas supply. As heat would destroy the valve it must be sterilised by ethylene oxide (p. 97).

(*b*) *The Ambu Hesse Valve.* Though similar in appearance to the Ruben Valve two elastic silicone shutters behave as unidirectional valves. It has the advantage that it can easily be dismantled for cleaning or sterilisation. Hot soapy water is suitable for cleansing.

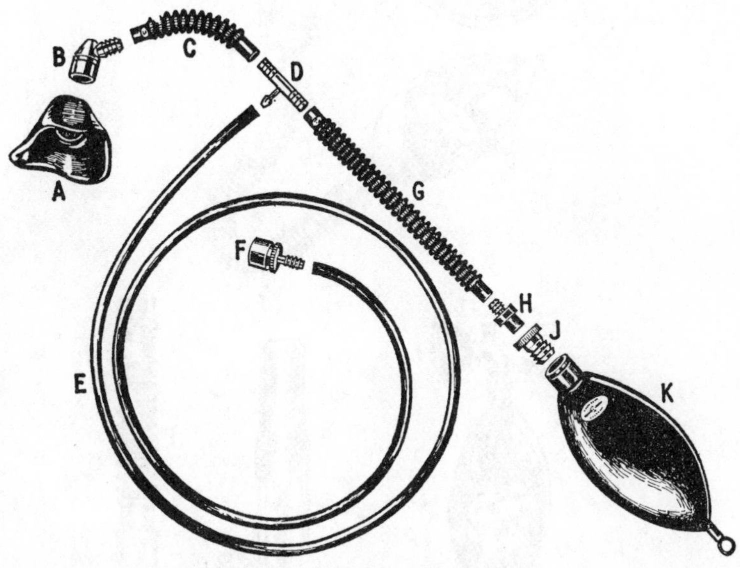

Fig. 38 'Open' paediatric set

The paediatric set is normally used without the reservoir bag. For endotracheal techniques, the face mask (A) and face mask adaptor (B) are removed and an endotracheal tube and connector substituted.

A Rendell-Baker face mask
B Face mask adaptor
C Corrugated tube
D Ayre's 'T' piece
E Supply tube
F Tubing mount
G Corrugated tube
H Hard rubber mount
J Bag adaptor
K Rebreathing bag 1 litre

Sterilisation can be carried out with most disinfectants (except phenol derivatives, ether or acetone) or hot air at temperatures of less than 120° C. Steam sterilisation under pressure is practicable but shortens the life of the silicone shutters.

(*c*) *The East Freeman Unidirectional Valve* is metal, but light in weight and not harmed by boiling or the high pressure autoclave.

(iii) Ayre's 'T' piece (Fig. 37). Introduced by Dr P. Ayre of

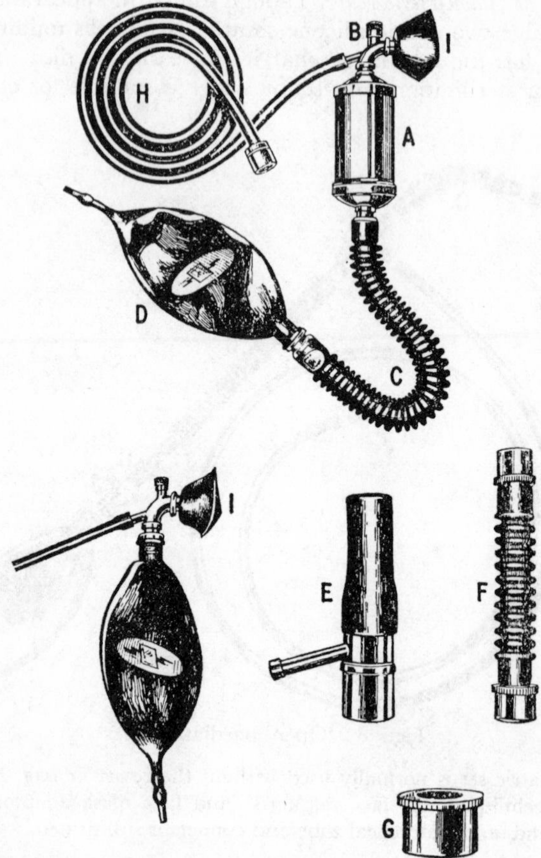

Fig. 39 Paediatric set for carbon dioxide absorption

A 85 g clear canister with caps
B curved face mask connector with expiratory valve
C corrugated extension piece
D latex bag with mount and vulcanite tap
E endotracheal connector with gas feed inlet
F flexible face mask connector
G child face mask adaptor for standard face masks
H feed tubing and mount
I Rendell-Baker Souchek infant's face mask

Newcastle many years ago, Ayre's 'T' piece is a small piece of 'T' shaped metal tubing whose *horizontal* limbs are longer and of slightly bigger diameter than the vertical limb which connects to the gas supply of the anaesthetic apparatus. One end of the horizontal limb carries an endotracheal tube and the other a short length of rubber tubing which serves as a rebreathing bag. The Ayre's 'T' piece is the simplest method of reducing resistance to respiration in paediatric anaesthesia and the principle is used in Magill's endotracheal tubes for infants (see below).

(iv) Endotracheal Tubes for paediatric anaesthesia are intended (*a*) to reduce resistance to breathing e.g. Cole's or Riplex tubes or (*b*) to reduce rebreathing to a minimum e.g. Magill's tubes.

(These tubes are illustrated and described more fully on page 63).

'Paediatric Sets.' Paediatric sets consists of an assembly of everything necessary for paediatric anaesthesia packed in a box and ready for use at any time.

There are two kinds in general use. One contains attachments for anaesthesia by the 'semi-open' method only and the other has additional equipment for 'To and Fro' carbon dioxide absorption. *The 'open' set* is assembled around an Ayre's 'T' piece with separate attachments for anaesthesia with a face mask or endotracheal tube. The essential components are to be seen in Fig. 38. *The carbon dioxide absorption set* has a curved face mask connector incorporating an expiratory valve; gas feed inlet, and a mount for a small Waters' canister and a rebreathing bag. *For endotracheal anaesthesia* there is a separate mount with gas feed inlet at the side which joins the tube and serves the same purpose as an Ayre's 'T' piece.

Note. The face masks of the carbon dioxide absorption set (Rendell-Baker Souchek) have a diameter less than that of a standard (Rendell-Baker) infant's face mask. A special adaptor (Fig. 39) is provided should a standard mask be needed. Being small it is easily mislaid.

7 THE ANAESTHETIC ROOM—IV

1. EQUIPMENT FOR INTRAVENOUS ANAESTHESIA

Equipment for intravenous anaesthesia is simple and consists of (i) syringes; (ii) hypodermic needles; and (iii) filling needles.

(i) Syringes. Syringes may be 'disposable' (sterilised by gamma radiation), or non-disposable, packed and sterilised in an autoclave by the C.S.S.D. or by a Syringe Service. Four sizes are in common use: 2 ml, 5 ml, 10 ml, and 20 ml.

(ii) Hypodermic Needles. Disposable hypodermic needles have replaced non-disposable needles which are difficult to clean properly and need re-sharpening before sterilisation. Besides ensuring absolute sterility and cleanliness, disposable needles spare the patient the discomfort of receiving an injection from a blunt-pointed needle. There are four sizes, distinguished by the colour of the cap of the plastic container or the plastic hub of the needle.

Dark Green indicates a number 1 needle—the largest size.
Pale Green or very Pale Blue indicates a number 12 needle—medium size.
Light Green indicates a number 17 needle—small size.
Blue or Orange indicates a number 20 needle—smallest size.

Note. It is *not necessary* to put a needle on every syringe, because (*a*) it may not be the size required, (*b*) the contents of two syringes are often injected through the same needle.

(iii) Filling Needle. A 'Filling needle' is a long (7·5 cm) large-bore needle used for mixing intravenous anaesthetics. Metal and disposable types are available.

2. NEEDLES FOR INTERMITTENT INTRAVENOUS INJECTIONS

It is often necessary to make repeated intravenous injections during anaesthesia. If an intravenous infusion (p. 79) is running, the rubber at the end of the infusion tubing can be used for this purpose. Otherwise, needles specially designed for intermittent injection (the Gordh or the Mitchell needle), are used, since a hypodermic needle left in a vein soon becomes blocked.

The Gordh Needle (Fig. 40a) has a transverse flange near the hub which carries a screw cap holding a small rubber diaphragm in position through which to make injections. A small quantity of injected fluid remains in the needle preventing the entry of blood and formation of a clot. When the needle is inserted, any blood which

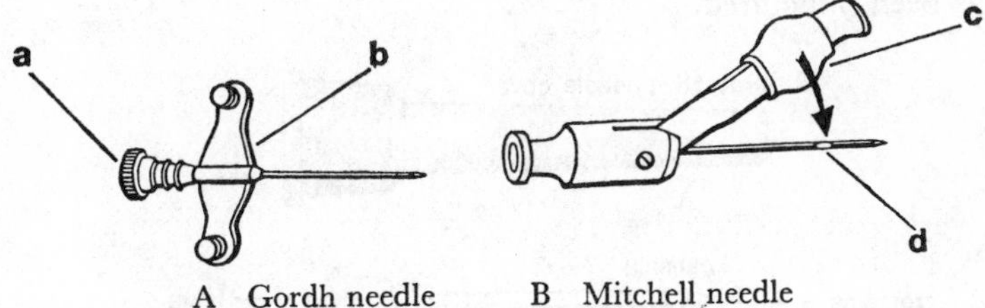

A Gordh needle B Mitchell needle

Fig. 40 Needles for intermittent intravenous injection

a screw cap and rubber diaphragm
b flange for fixation with tape or rubber band
c soft rubber cushion on movable arm secures needle in vein and covers
d opening in top side of needle

may have entered should be flushed out with a syringe containing saline or sterile water. The transverse flange allows fixation of the needle with a strip of adhesive tape, or a rubber strap. Disposable Gordh needles in the form known as 'butterfly infusion set' consist of a thin walled siliconed needle (to ease puncture) with a short length of plastic tubing ending in a luer adapter and plastic cap. Firm fixation with Elastoplast is advisable. After use, *non-disposable Gordh needles* require sharpening, careful cleansing and change of diaphragm before re-sterilisation.

The Mitchell Needle is slightly stouter than the Gordh needle. The opening is about 1·0 cm from the tip which is solid. When inserted in a vein, reflux of blood is prevented by sliding over the hole of the small rubber pad at the end of a light flat metal spring hinged on the hub (Fig. 40b). Being non-disposable it needs careful cleaning and sharpening before re-sterilisation.

3. NEEDLES AND CANNULAE FOR CONTINUOUS INTRAVENOUS INFUSION

A large bore needle in a vein, though adequate for the infusion of a single bottle of saline or blood, is unsuitable for long term intravenous therapy because ultimately it will perforate the vein and the fluid will run into the tissues. The insertion of a blunt-ended cannula for long-term use involves incision of the skin and vein leaving a sore wound and ultimately, a scar. This disadvantage is overcome by use of cannulae which can be inserted into a vein without incising the skin.

Cannulae are either (*a*) non-disposable or (*b*) disposable.

(*a*) Non-disposable cannulae are: *the Guest*, *the Frankis Evans*, and *West Middlesex patterns*. The West Middlesex cannula contains a *solid* needle, which must be withdrawn to ascertain whether the vein has been punctured.

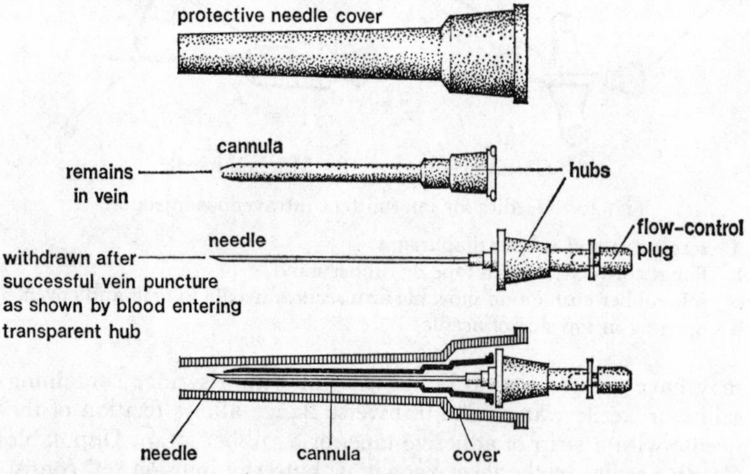

Fig. 41 Disposable needle intravenous cannula

(*b*) Disposable cannulae. The underlying principle of all types is the same. A sharp-pointed hollow needle passes *through* a plastic or metal cannula to just beyond its tip around which it fits snugly and smoothly. The needle carrying the cannula is inserted into a vein through the skin. The cannula enters the vein with the needle. Successful puncture is apparent when blood flows through the open end of the needle, or into a syringe which may have been fastened to it. The needle can then be withdrawn and the cannula attached to the infusion tubing and secured with adhesive tape.

(*b*) Disposable needles and cannulae. The '*Braunule*', '*Bardic around needle*' and '*Portex*' cannulae embody the principle already described. A transparent cap over the end of the needle serves as a 'trap' into which blood flows when the needle has entered the

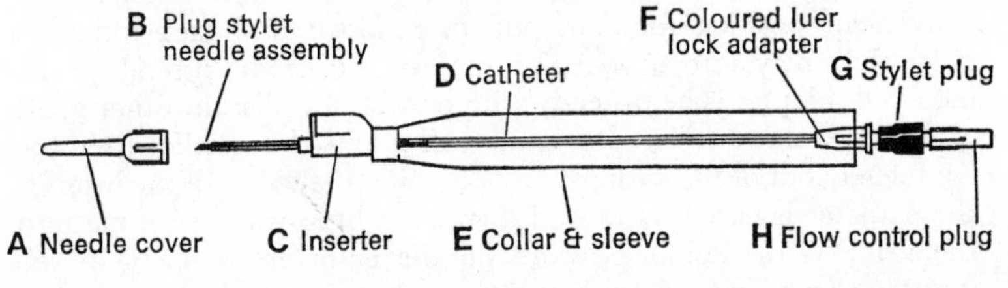

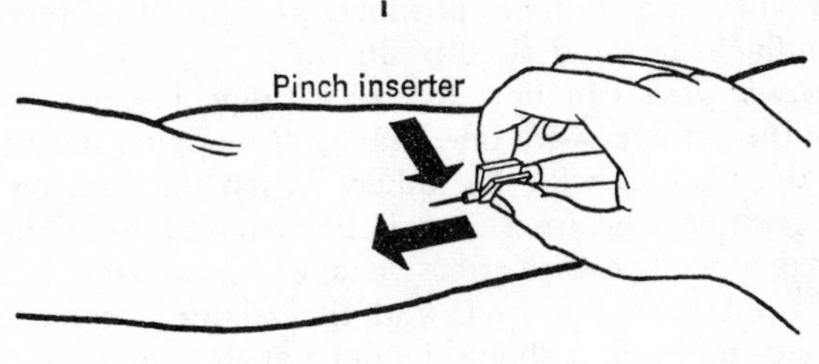

Fig. 42 A. Needle cover to be removed before use. B. Plug stylet needle assembly. C. Winged inserter which can be pinched between thumb and index fingers to secure needle and catheter. D. Catheter. E. Collar and transparent sleeve. F. Coloured luer lock adapter. G. Black stylet plug. S. Flow control plug.

vein. A disposable Guest cannula is also available. There is no blood trap but a 2 ml syringe placed on the hub serves the same purpose.

Making the cannula secure. Once the cannula has been successfully inserted, it must be secured to avoid withdrawal of the cannula by tension on the infusion tubing, and to prevent movement of the cannula within the vein. It should be secured and the puncture wound protected by a strip of 7·5 cm Elastoplast. The infusion tubing should then be looped backed on itself and fixed with a piece of 2·5 cm adhesive tape.

The Deseret E–Z Cath provides a method of inserting a nylon catheter into a vein without puncturing the skin, and providing proper aseptic precautions are taken reduces the incidences of complications arising from infection. The principle resembles that described already for intravenous cannulae but as the nylon catheter is flexible and longer than the plastic cannulae a plastic winged inserter is included (see fig. 42), which, on pinching between the thumb and index fingers can hold the needle and catheter in a convenient position for vein puncture. Blood flashback indicates successful entry into a vein. To remove the needle assembly, the coloured adapter is held steady with one hand whilst the other hand grasps the black stylet plug and withdraws the needle assembly completely out of the catheter. By pinching the wings of the inserter the catheter is carefully moved forward a little way at a time into the vein. With digital pressure on the catheter in the vein the inserter can be moved back a small distance and a further length inserted on release of digital pressure. This process is repeated until the cannulae is in the desired position.

The plastic sleeve can be removed by pinching the inserter and securing the catheter with one hand and snapping it away directly behind the adapter with the other. When the catheter is in the desired position, the inserter can be removed from the catheter which is then secured with adhesive tape and bandage. If the control plug has not been removed, and the adapter connected to the intravenous infusion, it should be done at this point.

4. CUT-DOWN SETS

Pre-packed sterile 'cut-down' sets are used to insert a cannula or nylon catheter if direct vein puncture is not possible.

The cut-down set should contain the following:

(i) Scalpel handle and small Bard Parker blade.
(ii) Two pairs of mosquito forceps.
(iii) Small cutting needles and fine catgut.
(iv) Small gauze swabs.
(v) Non-toothed dissecting forceps.
(vi) Nylon catheters, large and small diameters.
(vii) A Hamilton Bailey cannula. This cannula is of metal with a dinner fork bend and blunt rounded tip for ease of insertion into the vein. The opening of the cannula is a little behind the tip, whilst further back still, a raised ridge prevents the cannula slipping out of the vein until secured by catgut sutures passed through the holes in the flange on the hub (Fig. 43).

Scalp or small Vein Needle. A scalp or small vein needle is intended for insertion into the small veins of infants. It consists of a fine flanged needle, attached to a small-bore nylon tubing expanded at one end to take a Luer syringe or giving set. The needle needs careful fixation after insertion by adhesive tape placed over the flange. There are two sizes—21 swg and 23 swg × 2 cm long, packed in a gamma-ray sterilised plastic envelope.

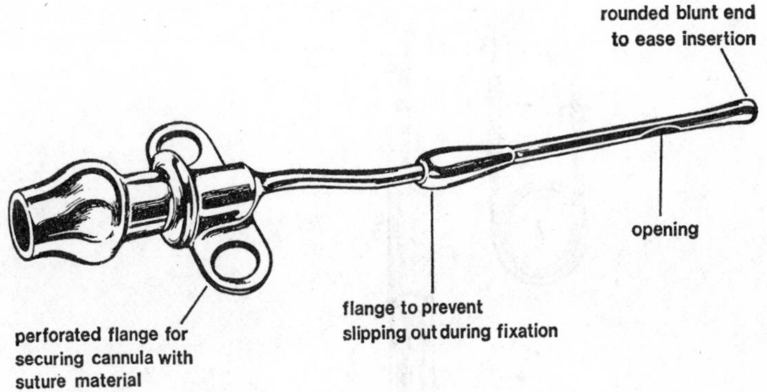

Fig. 43 Hamilton Bailey cannula

5. EQUIPMENT FOR ADMINISTRATION OF INTRAVENOUS FLUIDS

Sterile disposable apparatus for intravenous infusions ('giving sets') is now in universal use. There are two varieties, the *Baxter* and the *Capon Heaton*. They consist of:

(i) A sharp-pointed 'connector' to insert into the bottle (of fluid or blood) connected to

(ii) *A combined filter chamber and a drip device*, with a length of plastic tubing, ending a short length of rubber tubing (for injection purposes) and a nozzle for the intravenous cannula or needle.

(iii) *A screw clamp* on the tubing which controls the rate of flow.

(iv) *An air inlet.* Fluid will not run from a bottle unless air can enter to replace it. The Capon Heaton set has an air inlet incorporated in the drip chamber. The Baxter set has a separate length of tubing with a needle for this purpose.

The Baxter pressure pump (Fig. 44). The Baxter blood transfusion set has an ingenious pressure pump below the drip chamber. It is about 10 centimetres long and contains a white ball which floats on top of the fluid. Intermittent squeezing of the chamber with the flow control closed, draws blood from the bottle until the chamber is full, when the ball occludes the inlet. The flow control is then opened and further squeezing drives the blood onwards, the chamber refilling on release of pressure, and further squeezing pushes the ball up again and drives the blood onwards once more.

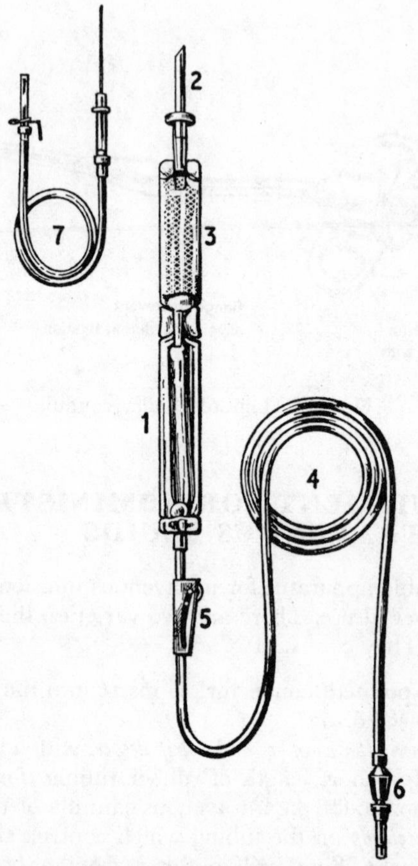

Fig. 44 Baxter blood administration set and pressure pump

1 pump chamber—cannot pump air
2 connector fits all types of blood and solution containers
3 seamless nylon fitter
4 delivery tubing
5 clamp which enables flow to be stopped
6 injection site
7 air inlet

Note. Plastic bottles require no air inlet because their sides collapse as the fluid runs out.

6. TYPES OF FLUID FOR INTRAVENOUS THERAPY

Fluids for intravenous therapy are:

(i) *Watery* solutions of *salts and sugars*.
(ii) *Watery* solutions of starchy substances known as *dextrans*.
(iii) *Dried* plasma (with sterile water for reconstitution).
(iv) *Whole blood.*
(v) *Hypertonic urea* solutions.

(i) Solutions of Salts and Sugars

(*a*) *Isotonic or 'Normal' Saline. 'Normal'* saline contains 9 g of salt per litre. It is 'isotonic' with body fluids. That is to say it does not attract water from the tissues (hypertonicity) nor will water pass from it to the tissues except by the normal process of filtration. Unless the patient is short of salt (e.g. from vomiting, diarrhoea, haemorrhage or excessive sweating), it is used sparingly. The body only needs 15 g of salt per day. Although the normal subject has no difficulty in excreting excess salt, this facility is impaired after surgery. Excessive salt intake is accompanied by fluid retention to maintain isotonicity of body fluids with 'waterlogging' (oedema) of the tissues, particularly when urine production is depressed after surgery. Normal saline is also used to flush out the giving-set before and after blood transfusion, because solutions containing glucose (see below) cause aggregation of red blood cells and may block the filter chamber.

(*b*) *Glucose Saline or '$\frac{1}{5}$ Normal' Saline.* Glucose saline contains 0·18% sodium chloride and 4·3% glucose, which ensures isotonicity although the salt content is $\frac{1}{5}$ that of 'Normal' saline. It provides salt, water and energy (Glucose) for patients who cannot take oral fluids.

(*c*) *5% Glucose in Water.* 5% Glucose solutions also provide a source of energy and protect the liver cells against toxic substances. The high glucose content is slightly irritant and can cause venous thrombosis after prolonged infusion whilst the absence of salt can give rise to 'water intoxication'; a disturbance of the central nervous system set up by passage of water into the brain cells because their salt content is higher than that of diluted plasma.

(*d*) *Ringer's Solution and Lactated Ringer's (Hartmann's) Solution*, are sometimes referred to as 'balanced' salt solutions because in addition to sodium chloride, they contain salts of potassium and calcium, all being of the same concentration as plasma. Hartmann's solution also contains sodium lactate. They have a reputation for maintaining the circulation in haemorrhage and traumatic shock, when blood is not available.

(*e*) *Mannitol 5% and 10%*. Mannitol is a carbohydrate (sugary) substance which, in contrast to glucose, is excreted by the kidney, carrying with it water which would otherwise have been absorbed back into the circulation. It is used to stimulate production of urine during and after major surgery.

(ii) Dextran Solutions. Although solutions of salts and sugars are useful to correct deficiencies in salts and water and to *maintain fluid balance*, their ability to support the circulation after haemorrhage and in shock states is limited, since more than half leaves the circulation and passes into the tissues, after about 1 to 1½ hours. *Dextrans* are starchy substances produced by fermentation of sugars with large molecules which remain in the circulation for as long as 24 hours and hence are of more value for emergency treatment of haemorrhage or traumatic shock until blood becomes available.

Note. There are two rules to be remembered when dextran is to be administered:

(*a*) blood *must* be taken before setting up an infusion because the presence of dextran in the blood stream can give rise to inaccuracies in grouping and cross-matching.

(*b*) Dextran is excreted by the kidney, and the large molecules can block the renal tubules and cause kidney damage. For this reason the quantity administered should be restricted to 1–2 litres in 24 hours. *Dextrans of low molecular weight* (dextran 40, see below) are less liable to cause trouble and may be used in larger quantities.

Solutions of dextran available for intravenous injection are:

Dextran 150/200:	average molecular weight 150,000 200,000	'Dextravan'
Dextran 110	,, ,, ,, 110,000	'Dextravan 100', 'Intradex'
Dextran 70	,, ,, ,, 70,000	'Macrodex'
Dextran 40	,, ,, ,, 40,000	'Rheomacrodex' 'Lomodex' 'Intraflodex'.

(iii) Dried Plasma. Dried plasma is prepared from blood whose corpuscles have become unsuitable for transfusion because of age or exposure to high temperatures. It is supplied in 500 ml bottles and can be reconstituted by addition of 500 ml of pyrogen-free sterile distilled water. Plasma is used for treatment of haemorrhagic or traumatic shock when blood is not available (e.g. war wounds or disasters), and is a specific indication for treatment of burns to compensate for loss of proteins in the serous oozing from burnt areas.

(iv) Whole Blood. Blood for transfusion is kept in a 'blood refrigerator' constructed to maintain a constant temperature between 4° and 6° Celsius. Domestic refrigerators are not suitable: if the temperature of the blood falls below 4°, it will freeze and the red cells will be destroyed (Haemolysis). Exposure to room temperature for *more than half an hour* with *subsequent* cooling in a refrigerator also destroys red cells. Blood should therefore remain in the refrigerator until needed. Although it will be cold when given, at normal flow rates it becomes sufficiently warm during passage down the transfusion tubing, but during rapid transfusion some method of warming the blood is necessary (see below).

Hazards of rapid massive transfusion. Rapid transfusion of more than two bottles of blood involves a risk of cardiac arrest (*a*) from cooling of the body to 29° C, or (*b*) from deficiency of 'ionised' calcium (essential for contraction of heart muscle) which is changed to an 'unionised' form by acid sodium citrate, added to blood to prevent clotting.

During massive transfusions (*a*) blood should be warmed by passage through a disposable heat conductive 'exchange coil' placed in a water bath kept at a constant temperature by a thermostatically controlled heater. Passage through an extension tubing immersed in a bucket of hot water is an effective but cumbersome and less accurate alternative method. (*b*) *Ionised calcium* in the form of calcium chloride or gluconate, 10 ml of a 5% solution should be given when more than two bottles of blood are given rapidly.

Checking Blood. Care should be taken to ensure that the patient receives the correct blood. If blood is not compatible, antibodies in the recipient's blood 'reject' and dissolve the foreign red cells, releasing large quantities of haemoglobin in the blood stream which block the kidneys and cause renal failure. *Partial incompatibility* can give rise to high fever and jaundice, a condition known as a 'transfusion reaction'.

To avoid mistakes when checking the blood bottle, the pathologist's report, the patient's notes, and his identity band should be examined to confirm that the patient's *name*, *hospital number*, *ward*, *blood group*, and *number of the bottle* coincide. Mistakes have arisen when two people with similar names have had blood prepared; also on other occasions blood has been checked against the *notes of another patient*—hence the importance of ensuring that patient's record sheet and the patient's identity band coincide.

(v) Urea for injection. Solutions of urea dissolved in hypertonic dextrose are used to reduce cerebral oedema resulting from head injuries or during operations on the brain. The 'hypertonic' solution draws water from the tissues. The solution should be freshly prepared by mixing 40 mg of urea with 105 ml of 5 or 10% dextrose.

8 THE ANAESTHETIC ROOM—V

MONITORING EQUIPMENT

The observation and recording of cardiac and respiratory function is known as '*monitoring*'. Although the word monitor has traditionally an admonitory or disciplinary sense it also implies '*supervision*'. The anaesthetic room contains several items of equipment for this purpose. These are for: (i) Measurement of *blood pressure.* (ii) Measurement of *venous pressure.* (iii) Recording of the *pulse.* (iv) Recording the *electrical activity of the heart* (electrocardiograph). (v) For observing *carbon dioxide content of inspired or expired gases.* (vi) To assess *respiratory function* (respirometer). (vii) To measure *blood loss* during surgery.

(i) Measurement of blood pressure. Measurement of blood pressure is a routine procedure during anaesthesia for major surgery. The pressure cuff and brachial stethoscope should be applied to the patient's arm *after* induction of anaesthesia (p. 94). For convenience the sphygmomanometer, either aneroid (dial type) or mercurial is often fixed to a bracket on the anaesthetic apparatus.

An *oscillotonometer* is an aneroid sphygmomanometer in which the oscillations of the needle set up by the arterial pulsations can be magnified by moving a small lever. Measurements of systolic and diastolic blood pressure is possible by observation of the needle's oscillations thus making use of a brachial stethoscope unnecessary. The instrument is easily damaged if dropped and should be permanently secured to a bracket on the anaesthetic apparatus.

(ii) Measurement of venous pressure. Measurement of venous pressure is not a routine procedure. It is used during operations associated with shock and haemorrhage; or for patients under treatment for traumatic or septic shock. Venous pressure is measured by passing a nylon catheter through an arm or neck vein, into the superior vena cava and connecting it to a water manometer. Disposable apparatus is available for this purpose. It consists of a disposable intravenous set to which (Fig. 45) a plastic three-way 'Y' piece (B) with tap is attached. One branch (C) of the 'Y' connects to the vein, one (D) to a bottle of saline, and the third (A) to a vertical tube and manometer scale. The zero point on the scale should be

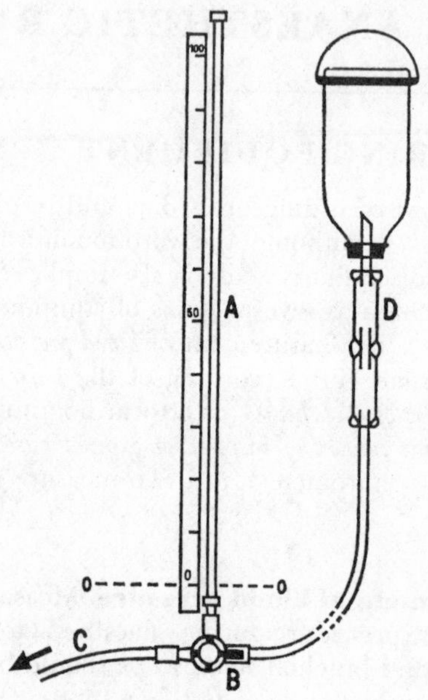

Fig. 45 Principle of venous pressure measurement

A manometer scale
B 3-way tap
C lead to patient's vein
D drip chamber and connector

adjusted to the level of the manubrium (the angle) of the sternum or to a mid-axillary line, both of which coincide with the level of the right auricle. *To measure the pressure*, the tube leading to the infusion bottle is *closed* and that to the *manometer* is *opened*. The level of fluid in the manometer indicates the pressure in the vein. The significance of venous pressure is discussed further on page 160.

(iii) Recording of the pulse (Pulsometers). Electrical apparatus for continuous recording of the pulse rate are known as pulse monitors or 'pulsometers', and consist of (*a*) a small microphone and lead which is attached to the finger tip and (*b*) a small box containing receiving and amplifying units. They record the pulse by means of a flashing light or buzzer and may include a dial to indicate the rate.

Pulsometers, besides providing a constant record of the pulse rate and of irregularities can also be used to measure systolic blood pressure when used in combination with sphygmomanometer and pressure cuff, systolic blood pressure coinciding with disappearance of the pulse record. The method is not thoroughly dependable because the microphone is easily dislodged from the finger (with disappearance of the record) and it is not always practicable to replace it. The great toe has been suggested as preferable to the finger since access is simpler.

Note. To monitor pulse and respiration in small infants, a diaphragm type of stethoscope strapped over the heart, or an earpiece connected to a fine plastic tube which is passed into the oesophagus provides a reliable audible record of the heart beat and respiration.

(iv) The Electrocardiograph records the electrical activity set up by the contraction of the heart muscle, following the passage of nervous impulses through the ventricles from the 'pacemaker' in the right auricle, either by means of a *cardioscope*, a small cathode ray oscilloscope, or by a 'writing device'.

The electrocardiograph or cardioscope is connected to the patient by electrodes known as 'leads'. There are three pairs. Each carries a cone for a hypodermic needle, which is inserted under the skin (after induction of anaesthesia) in the following way, Lead I—to right and left arm; Lead II—to right arm and left leg; Lead III—to left arm and left leg.

Continuous observation of the electrocardiogram is a means of detecting cardiac irregularities during anaesthesia and gives a continuous record of the pulse rate.

(v) Analysis of blood gases. During operations on the heart and blood vessels and especially during and after extra-corporeal perfusion ('pump cases'), repeated estimation of the oxygen and carbon dioxide tensions in the arterial blood are often necessary. An indirect way of doing this in conscious patients is to take samples of alveolar air, but during anaesthesia direct examination of arterial blood samples is necessary. Samples are taken at intervals from a fine catheter usually inserted into the radial artery because should this small artery become thrombosed or damaged during the process no permanent harm will follow. Indwelling catheters in arteries can also be used for direct measurement and recording of blood pressure.

Following removal of a needle or catheter from an artery firm pressure is required to ensure against leakage and formation of a haematoma.

(vi) The Wright Respirometer. This small instrument measures the volume of air expired at each breath. It is used at the end of the operation to assess the adequacy of respiration, especially if there is doubt whether the effects of muscle relaxants have worn off or to what extent respiration is depressed by opiates or anaesthesia. The respirometer is a small metal instrument, 63 mm by 55 mm with a watch face type dial with two scales. The larger measures the *volume* of each *expiration*, the smaller the *sum* of successive breaths for measurement of *minute volume.* On the outside of the dial there is (*a*) a spring loaded button which re-sets the hands of the dial to zero and (*b*) an 'on/off' control. When not in use the respirometer should be kept in a small black leather case which contains circular metal adaptors (Fig. 46) to allow insertion into any make of anaesthetic circuit.

The respirometer is a delicate instrument which should be handled with care. After use, a gentle current of air or oxygen should be blown through it for a few minutes to remove traces of water or anaesthetic vapour.

(vii) Measurement of Blood Loss. Measurement of blood lost during operation helps to assess the requirements for blood replacement. There are three methods:

(*a*) *Gravimetric* (Swab weighing). Swabs and packs are weighed before and after use and any increase in weight recorded. 1 mg of blood is equal to 1 ml of blood. When using this method an addition of up to 30% of the blood loss should be made to allow for blood not measured but spilt on towels and gowns or taken into the suction apparatus. The exact figure depends on the nature of the operation.

(*b*) *Colorimetric methods.* All swabs, towels and gowns are washed in a measured volume of water. The haemoglobin (in the red cells) is dissolved and the quantity calculated by comparison with a colour chart, from which the amount of blood loss is calculated. The haemoglobin value for the patient at the beginning of the operation must be available.

The Medatron Blood Loss Meter operates on the above principle the dissolved haemoglobin being measured by a photo-electric cell.

(*c*) *Measurement of Blood Volume.* Electronic computerised machines (e.g. the 'Volmetron') are manufactured to measure red cell volume by means of radioactive isotopes. The instrument records radioactivity of blood samples before and after a small intravenous

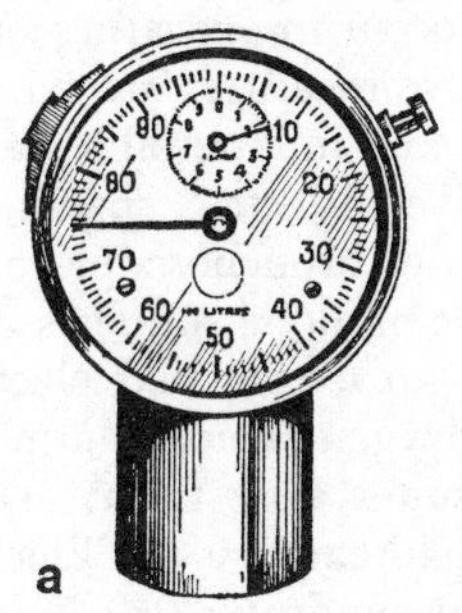

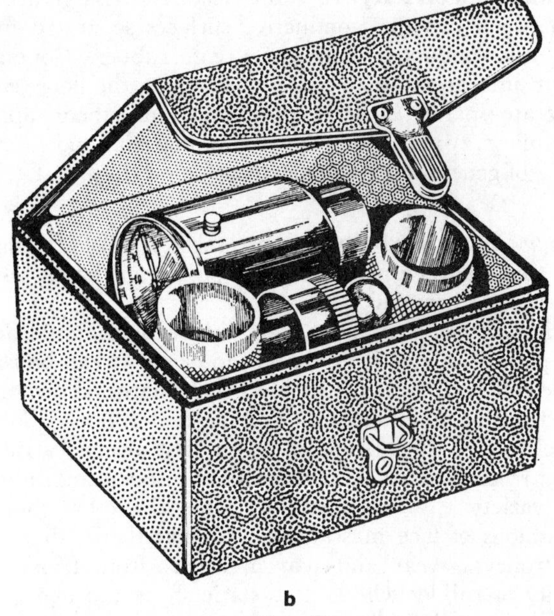

Fig. 46

a Wright respirometer b respirometer in case with adaptors

injection of radioactive substance, from which it calculates the blood volume and indicates it on the measuring scale. The method is easy and quick, and the dose of radioactive material harmless to the patient and those who handle it.

PREVENTION OF FIRE AND EXPLOSIONS

Fires or explosions may occur in operating suites for several reasons unless adequate preventive measures are taken.

Ether and cyclopropane are inflammable, and when mixed with oxygen become explosive. Electric sparks, or the intense heat generated by light bulbs of bronchoscopes or oesophagoscopes can cause a detonation. Oxygen alone supports combustion; smouldering material (e.g. from an overheated electrical connection) will burst into flames in an oxygen enriched atmosphere.

Sparks in operating suites arise from: (1) Static electricity. (2) Diathermy and the 'actual' cautery. (3) Electric plugs and connections. (4) Portable X-ray apparatus. (5) Faulty electrical contacts.

(1) Static electricity. A 'static' electrical charge arises from friction between two dry conductive surfaces separated from the earth by non-conductive substances e.g. rubber. Contact with similar but 'uncharged' material, or passage to the floor (earthing) may generate sparks. Theatre personnel, anaesthetic apparatus, dressing trolleys, woollen blankets, nylon material and formica are all capable of generating static electricity.

Preventive measures. Precautions are taken in all operating suites to ensure that static electrical charges pass immediately to 'earth' and are rendered harmless.

(i) *'Anti-static' rubber.* Rubber is an insulating material and prevents the passage of electrical charges to earth. It can be rendered conductive and will 'earth' any electrical charge if carbon is incorporated during manufacture. This type of rubber is known as 'anti-static' rubber. It is black in colour, but always carries a distinguishing *yellow marking.* All rubber used in operating suites must be of this variety, e.g. suction tubing; anaesthetic breathing hose; rubber cushions of face masks; tyres of anaesthetic, dressing and patients' trolleys. Wear and tear and wax from floors reduces conductivity of rubber wheels, anti-static shoes and boots, so that testing of their conductivity at regular intervals is recommended.

(ii) *Footwear* must be of anti-static rubber or have conductive soles of wood, rope or cotton. *Nylon shirts or underwear* should not be worn because static charges can arise in them from contact with the skin. Cotton material is non-conductive and more suitable for wear in operating suites. *Woollen blankets* must be replaced by cellular cotton blankets in the 'transfer zone'. Patients should wear cotton pyjamas or night gowns.

(iii) Formica arm retainers should have cotton covers.

(iv) *The floors* of anaesthetic rooms and operating theatres should be 'anti-static'.

(v) *Dry warm air* is favourable for generation of static charges and ventilating systems should ensure a flow of cool air at a *humidity of 70%*. Badly ventilated operating suites in which the heating system is left on overnight produce dry warm air favourable for static sparks. In these circumstances water poured on the floor and soaking the anaesthetic hoses in water before use will raise humidity sufficiently to avoid the generation of static charges.

(2) Diathermy produces sparks freely, and the 'actual cautery' red heat. When used the *ether bottle should be removed* from the apparatus, the cyclopropane cylinder closed, and the key removed.

(3) Electric plugs and connections. The switch mechanism of sockets generates sparks when contact is made or broken. The risk of explosion is avoided by placing sockets at least 120 cm above floor level, since anaesthetic gases are heavier than air and accumulate at floor level. Plugs at lower levels should be of a type which do not create sparks.

(4) Portable X-ray apparatus is capable of producing sparks if faults develop. When it is in use the precautions described for diathermy equipment should be observed.

(5) Faulty contacts or short circuits in electrical apparatus, especially electric suction equipment are a potential source of sparks. Regular inspection and maintenance of all electrical equipment used in the operating suite is the best insurance against accidents.

Other causes of fire. The presence of oil on reducing valves or cylinder nozzles can cause a fire if a leak develops. Lubricants should not be necessary with modern equipment, but should need arise, a non-greasy lubricant is available.

Compressed air in cylinders may be contaminated by fine particles of oil and may ignite in the presence of intense heat such as produced by a drill driven by compressed air.

9 THE ANAESTHETIC ROOM—VI

This chapter deals briefly with practical suggestions for the general layout of the anaesthetic room, together with points about routine preparations for anaesthesia, intubation, etc. and concludes with a discussion on the ways and means of cleansing and sterilising anaesthetic equipment.

ORGANISATION AND PREPARATIONS FOR ANAESTHESIA

General Lay-out. It is customary at present to keep in the anaesthetic room all equipment and apparatus (including ventilators and cardiac monitoring equipment) used for anaesthesia. Many items (e.g. endobronchial tubes, bronchoscopes) are not required frequently, whilst others (e.g. syringes, needles) are needed for every anaesthetic. Thought should therefore be given to storage; items in common use being kept in easily accessible positions whilst those less often needed can be put further away. Thus (especially in emergency) preparations for anaesthesia can be made quickly without delay involved in collecting missing items from around the room.

Syringes are constantly needed and a convenient method of storage is in a 'dispenser' placed on the wall above the work bench or trolley, which can be 'topped up' as needed from boxes of syringes kept in a cupboard away from the working area.

Needles. An assortment of needles can be kept in the lower compartment of the syringe dispenser.

Drugs. Some idea of the variety of drugs which an anaesthetic room may contain can be obtained from the therapeutic index (Chapter 22). In order that they can be found easily when needed, they should be stored according to their classification . . . e.g. 'vasopressors', 'relaxants', 'respiratory stimulants', etc. A selection of those in routine use should be kept on the bench or trolley in some form of dispenser made of wood or formica with groups of six holes labelled for ampoules. Such an arrangement saves time at the start of the day's work as well as when preparing for an emergency anaesthetic.

Endotracheal equipment. A *laryngoscope*, *Magill's forceps*, and *local anaesthetic spray* (p. 68) should be kept ready on the anaesthetic apparatus. *Endotracheal tubes* (p. 61) are stored according to size; *cuffed* and *plain* tubes should be in separate compartments of a drawer or cupboard but within easy reach. *Endotracheal connections* should be kept in sets, clearly labelled in boxes. A piece of wood or formica with cut-outs for each connection of a set is a useful method of storage and any missing connection soon becomes apparent. A *syringe to inflate cuffed tubes* and a clip (an old artery forceps) to close the inflating tube should also be kept on the top of the anaesthetic apparatus.

Intravenous infusions. *Disposable giving sets*, *intravenous fluids* and disposable *intravenous cannulae* may be required at short notice and should *not* be stored in a cupboard where access is difficult. It is a wise plan always to have a *giving set*; *I.V. fluid*, and a *cannula* ready for use near the anaesthetic apparatus.

Routine Checking of the Anaesthetic Machine

The apparatus should be checked before use so that any deficiencies, e.g. empty cylinders, can be corrected before the arrival of the patient.

(i) There should be no 'empty' cylinders. 'In use' cylinders should be open and ready for use. (This can be confirmed by opening the appropriate rotameter screw and seeing the bobbin rise in the tube.)

(ii) The 'full' cylinders should be closed.

(iii) The emergency oxygen tap should be tested.

(iv) The vaporising bottles (except the Fluothane vaporiser) should be empty. Normally they are emptied at the end of each day because whoever uses the apparatus next will not know for certain what they contain. Fluothane vaporisers, not being used for any other agent, are exempted from this rule.

(v) When diathermy is to be used, the cyclopropane cylinder closed and the key removed (p. 91).

(vi) A face-piece harness and means of fixing it should be on the machine.

(vii) The Magill attachment with an 'angle piece' and endotracheal adaptor and mount should be available.

(viii) Soda lime in the CO_2 absorber should be checked and hose and re-breathing bag in position.

(ix) The 'Bosun' warning device should be tested (p. 39).

(x) A clean cotton or disposable paper towel should be placed on the trolley top together with a receiver for soiled equipment (syringes, airways, laryngoscope).

INDUCTION OF ANAESTHESIA

The identity of the patient, the proposed operation and the pre-operative injection should be checked before the induction of anaesthesia. The presence of an assistant during induction and endotracheal intubation is essential.

Intravenous Induction

(i) The spotlight should be turned on and directed on to the patient's forearm.

(ii) The assistant should distend the veins of the arm by gentle compression with the hand (insufficient to obstruct the artery) above the elbow.

(iii) If the upper arm is too large or the hand too small to encompass it, the veins can be occluded by looping a finger in the sleeve of the patient's gown and twisting gently. At the same time the patient should be asked to open and close the fist in order to distend the veins still further.

(iv) If difficulty is experienced in finding a vein in the forearm, it may be possible to find one on the back of the hand. Some consider the veins on the back of the hand preferable to those of the forearm because risk of intra-arterial injection is less. Nevertheless, puncture on the back of the hand produces bruising which often gives rise to greater concern than the operation.

(v) Compression of the veins should continue until successful puncture has been made (shown by blood entering the syringe) and the anaesthetist gives a signal for release.

(vi) Thereafter the arm should be supported steadily until the injection is completed, because any slight movement at this stage can dislodge the needle causing subcutaneous injection.

(vii) If endotracheal intubation is to be carried out, a second injection of muscle relaxant through the same needle will follow the intravenous anaesthetic.

Endotracheal Intubation

During the passage of an endotracheal tube:

(i) The assistant should stand facing the anaesthetist and on the same side as the anaesthetic apparatus. It is helpful to hold the tube in one hand ready to pass to the anaesthetist when he has visualised the larynx.

(ii) If difficulty is experienced in seeing the larynx, help can be given:

(*a*) by pressing gently in an upward direction on the thyroid cartilage ('Adam's apple') which will bring the laryngeal opening upwards and forwards into the line of vision of the anaesthetist;

(*b*) by placing the forefinger inside the cheek and drawing it gently outwards on the same side as the laryngoscope (the laryngoscope is seldom passed exactly in the midline). This manœuvre pulls the base of the tongue sideways, flattening it and bringing the pharynx and larynx into the line of vision.

(iii) When the tube has been passed, the endotracheal mount and tube (p. 65) and anaesthetic hose should be handed to the anaesthetist.

(iv) The cuff should be inflated with the syringe and clipped off when inflation is judged adequate by the anaesthetist.

(v) Linen or adhesive tape will be needed to secure the anaesthetic hose and endotracheal mount to the patient and should be prepared beforehand.

(vi) If an intravenous infusion is required, it should be started before moving into the theatre.

Inhalational induction is rare except for children. When used, absolute silence is essential and the assistant should stand at the side of the patient facing the anaesthetist, ready to restrain the patient, gently but firmly, if necessary during the 'struggling' stage (uncommon except when using ether) which marks the transition from the conscious to the unconscious state. The concern of the anaesthetist at this stage is to keep the mask firmly on the patient's face because, after one or two breaths of air, consciousness will return and the induction must begin all over again.

Transfer to the operating theatre. After induction the *diathermy pad* and *blood pressure cuff* (p. 85) should be applied to *leg* and *arm. The eyes should be closed* and *sealed* with '*clear tape*' or covered by a *piece of tulle gras and a gauze eye pad.* When the anaesthetist gives the signal to move, theatre porters move the patient whilst the nurse or technician helps to move the anaesthetic machine so that it does not become separated from the patient.

Once the patient is transferred to the operating table the anaesthetist should have within reach any drugs or equipment required during the operation without having to leave the patient or call for assistance. This is best met by having a 'drug trolley' carrying any items needed, but if a trolley is not available, the top of the anaesthetic apparatus makes a less satisfactory alternative.

Suction apparatus with a supply of catheters and a bowl of water to clear the suction tubing after use should be available at all times.

The anaesthetic record should be taken from the patient's notes and placed on a 'clip board' for recording the progress of the anaesthetic.

When the needs of the anaesthetist have been met, attention should be directed to the anaesthetic room which should be tidied and made ready for the next patient. Used syringes should be removed, empty ampoules cleared away, and drugs replaced from store.

CLEANING AND STERILISATION OF ANAESTHETIC EQUIPMENT

Sterilisation of anaesthetic equipment and apparatus is necessary to prevent infection passing from patient to patient ('cross infection'). Every piece of equipment which comes into contact with a patient collects bacteria. Although many are not harmful, a small proportion can cause serious infection if they pass to another patient. There is no standard procedure for sterilisation of anaesthetic equipment and apparatus. Practice depends on the facilities available at different hospitals, and the scope and extent of the C.S.S.D. Any of the methods described below are acceptable.

(1) Sterilisation by Heat

(i) *Boiling for fifteen minutes* will destroy bacteria, although repeated boiling destroys rubber and plastic material.

(ii) *Pasteurisation*—exposure to 75° C for 10 minutes destroys all pathogenic bacteria and is an acceptable alternative for materials which are damaged by high temperature. A thermostatically controlled water bath at 75° C is suitable for sterilising face masks, laryngoscope blades, airways, endotracheal tubes and connections.

(iii) *Autoclave sterilisation.* In an autoclave, steam under pressure of 15 lb per sq. in. reaches a temperature of 120° C, sufficient to destroy all bacteria and spores of anaerobic bacilli (e.g. *clostridium welchii* which causes gas gangrene). Rubber also deteriorates under this treatment and sharp instruments become blunted and there is no necessity to destroy spores. Small 'low pressure' autoclaves are less destructive and are used increasingly in Recovery Rooms and Anaesthetic Rooms to sterilise small items of equipment like endotracheal connections, laryngoscope blades, airways, and endotracheal mounts.

(2) Chemical Sterilisation

Several disinfectants are available. Some in common use are:

(i) *Ethylene oxide*—a colourless gas, has excellent disinfectant properties but is slow in action (8–12 hours) and highly inflammable; a risk that can be decreased by mixture with 90% carbon dioxide. Sterilisation of ventilators, respirometers and Ruben's valves (p. 70) are best carried out by this method since exposure to an autoclave would ruin these instruments. Sterilisation can be accomplished by sealing the instrument in a transparent bag filled with the gas. Ethylene oxide sterilisers are expensive but sharing by several hospitals reduces the overall cost. A high-speed nebuliser has been introduced for sterilisation of ventilators.

(ii) *Liquid chemical disinfectants* are too numerous to mention in detail. Those suitable for anaesthetic equipment are: (*a*) *Ethyl alcohol 75%*; whilst not a complete disinfectant it is useful when quick cleansing is required and for 'damp dusting' apparatus, etc. (*b*) *Chlorhexidine 1% aqueous solution* ('Hibitane') sterilises in about half an hour. Unfortunately it tends to make rubber 'sticky'. (*c*) *Activated glutaraldehyde* ('Cidex') sterilises thoroughly and retains its activity for two or more weeks and resists inactivation by detergents. It is irritant to the skin and needs careful handling. Its vapour is rather unpleasant so that containers should be kept sealed.

Suggested Methods for Cleaning and Disinfecting Various Items

The method for cleaning and disinfecting various items of anaesthetic equipment will naturally vary with the facilities available at the hospital concerned. The following suggestions are the simplest which can be safely carried out.

Endotracheal tubes and connections; face masks; suction catheters; laryngoscope blades and oral airways should be washed in warm water and soap after use. Care is necessary to clean the *inside* of tubes and airways with test tube brushes. They can then be placed in chlorhexidine 1% for half an hour, then rinsed again and dried, or pasteurised in a water bath. At this stage they are ready for use again. An alternative and more sophisticated method is by wrapping in paper or cellophane and passage through a low-pressure autoclave.

Corrugated re-breathing tubes and reservoir bags should be washed each day after use and hung up to dry. Once a week they should be immersed in 1 % chlorhexidine for an hour. Pasteurisation in a low pressure autoclave is satisfactory and does not destroy the anti-static properties of the rubber.

Waters' canisters can easily be sterilised by boiling or in an autoclave.

Circle absorbers can be sterilised with ethylene oxide at intervals or dismantled and cleaned with 75 % alcohol or 1 % chlorhexidine.

Note. When any apparatus or equipment is used for a patient known to be suffering from *'open' tuberculosis* (i.e. with tubercle bacilla in the sputum) or from *pyocyaneus infection*, it should be withdrawn for sterilisation in a high-pressure autoclave or, if unsuitable for autoclaving, by ethylene oxide.

10 POSITION OF THE PATIENT ON THE OPERATING TABLE

GENERAL RULES

Before discussing details about positions of the patient on the operating table, there are some general rules which apply in every instance.

1. The patient should always be covered, as far as possible, particularly at the *end* of an operation.

2. An unconscious patient is insensitive to pain, for this reason constant care is needed to avoid injury during movement and positioning. For example:

(i) *Joints* may be injured. Arthritic patients often have restricted movements. Joints should never be *forced.*

(ii) *Nerves* may be damaged from pressure or stretching. *Pressure* on the nerve at the *outer side of the knee* (peroneal) or the nerve that winds round the *back of the arm* (radial) can cause paralysis of ankle or wrist joints ('*foot drop*' or '*wrist drop*'). *Stretching* of the nerve trunks of the *brachial plexus* can cause paralysis of the arm or shoulder; a risk much increased when the arm is put at right angles to the body in the 'head down' (Trendelenberg) position.

(iii) *Blood vessels.* (*a*) *veins.* If subject to pressure, thrombosis occurs causing obstruction. (*b*) Following damage to an artery (e.g. popliteal behind the knee) spasm and thrombosis can cause gangrene.

(iv) The skin should be protected from heat and abrasion. When diathermy is being used no skin should come into contact with the metal of the operating table, since burns may result from the diathermy current 'shorting' to earth through the table.

COMMON POSITIONS FOR SURGERY

The common positions for surgery are: 1. *Supine.* 2. *Trendelenberg.* 3. *Lithotomy.* 4. *Lateral.* 5. *Prone.*

(1) The Supine position. In the supine position, the patient lies on the back with the arms either at the side or flexed on the chest. If at the side, they should be secured by a towel or arm holder to prevent the arm slipping over the side of the table during the operation, damaging the *radial* (see above) or *ulnar nerve*. It may be necessary to have one arm supported in an abducted position for intravenous therapy. A well-padded arm rest should support the arm, which should be placed with the palm downwards, whilst the angle with the body should be *less than a* right angle to avoid stretching the brachial plexus. Whenever possible, both arms should be at the side or flexed on the chest, for if there is more than one surgical assistant there is a constant danger of the arm being forced upwards in attempts to gain access to the operating area.

The heels should be supported by padded hollow rings thus reducing the risk of venous thrombosis by taking the weight of the legs off the calves.

(2) The Trendelenberg position is a variation of the supine position used to improve access to the pelvis. (Gynaecological and genito-urinary operations and surgery of the sigmoid colon.) The patient lies on his back with the table tilted so that the head points towards the floor and the legs towards the ceiling. Steps must be taken to prevent the patient sliding off the table: (*a*) by the use of a ridged non-slip mattress on which the patient should lie without the intervention of a drawsheet. (*b*) If a non-slip mattress is not available, shoulder rests which fit into the top of the table are used. They should be well padded and placed to support the *outer* part of the shoulder (acromioclavicular joint), to avoid pressure on the nerves of the brachial plexus on the inner side.

Note. Abduction of the arm in the Trendelenberg position carries a greater risk of damage to the brachial plexus than when the patient is flat.

(3) The Lithotomy position—so-called from medieval times when it was used in the operation for removal of stones in the bladder ('cutting for stone') via the perineum. The lithotomy position is required for *operations* on the vagina; the urethra; the anus and rectum, and for *examinations* of the bladder (cystoscopy); the rectum (proctoscopy); and the sigmoid colon (sigmoidoscopy).

Both legs are lifted off the table and abducted to an angle of 45 degrees. The knees are flexed and the feet are secured in a sling hung from two upright rods at the side of the table. The patient is put in this position in the following way: (i) The buttocks are placed over the break at the end of the table, which is let down or removed to allow access to the perineum. (ii) The leg supports, with the foot slings already in place, are placed in position. Both supports should be at exactly the same level and their *height* equal to the *length of the patient's thighs.* (iii) The legs are raised simultaneously by the assistants to approximately 45 degrees, when the knees are flexed with one hand on the thigh and one on the leg. The foot is moved *outside* the support and fixed in the canvas sling—one band round the foot and the other round the lower end of the calf. (Some find this procedure difficult and it should be studied beforehand.) Simultaneous raising of the legs avoids strain of the sacro-iliac joints. Movement should never be *forced*; resistance to flexion suggests a possibility of arthritic changes in the hip joint, the leg should be held by an assistant throughout the operation. When the feet are anchored in the slings care should be taken to make sure that no skin comes into contact with the metal of the support, which is padded in its upper half to avoid this. Pressure on the calf muscles and the nerve on the outer side of the leg is prevented by adjusting the supports and by generous padding.

At the end of the operation the foot of the table is raised or replaced and the legs lowered simultaneously by two assistants. The legs being supported until the end of the table has been replaced.

The arms are folded over the chest and tucked into the operation gown.

(4) The Lateral (Nephrectomy) position is used for operations on the *chest* (Thoracotomy), the *kidney* (Nephrectomy), and the *spinal column* (Laminectomy). The prone position may also be used for this last operation.

In this position the trunk tends to roll forwards or backwards; pressure on nerves and blood vessels in the dependent arm and stretching of the nerves and joints of the upper arm is a constant hazard.

Lateral position for nephrectomy. The steps for placing the patient in position are: (i) The '*kidney bridge*' in the centre of the operating table is located and the patient transferred to the operating table, with the loin directly over it. (ii) The *patient is turned on to the side.* Three people should assist: the anaesthetist controls the head; one assistant controls the trunk; another the pelvis and legs. When in the lateral position, one assistant should hold the patient until the pelvis and trunk are stabilised. (iii) *The pelvis is stabilised* (*a*) by flexing the *dependent* leg at the *hip* and *knee*, leaving the *uppermost* leg straight. A pillow or rubber pad is placed between the knees. (*b*) Passing a strip of Elastoplast or strap over the pelvis at the level of the great trochanter and securing it firmly at each side of the operating table. (iv) *Stabilisation of the trunk* is achieved (*a*) by an arm rest (Carter Braine) fixed to the table in front of the patient, on which the elbow and forearm are placed. The elbow may be flexed or extended, until the shoulder is in line with the hip, when the forearm and wrist should be bandaged to the support with the interposition of ample gauze tissue, and (*b*) by placing a sandbag along the back and a padded support against the front of the chest. (c) The lower arm should be drawn forward from under the patient and gently flexed or placed on an arm board, to reduce venous obstruction from the weight of the body on the lower arm.

The kidney bridge is then raised. If the patient has been correctly positioned, the site of operation will be elevated and the space between the ribs and crest of the iliac bone will be widened, offering good access to the kidney region.

If the lateral position is required to open the *chest* or upper abdomen, the kidney bridge is not necessary. The surgeon's exact requirements should always be ascertained beforehand.

(5) The Prone position. The patient lies face downwards. Before turning the patient, two pillows or sandbags should be ready to place under the chest and the pelvis after turning, to prevent embarrassment of respiration in an unconscious subject by the weight of the body compressing the abdomen thus preventing descent of the diaphragm and expansion of the chest.

Before the turning of the patient, the anaesthetic apparatus is disconnected until the turn has been completed. If an intravenous infusion has been set up, it should also be disconnected during the turning process.

To turn the patient two assistants are necessary. The anaesthetist takes care of the head and shoulders, one assistant holds the chest and arms and one the pelvis and legs. There are three movements involved: (i) The assistants draw the patient towards one side of the table, supporting chest and pelvis. (ii) The patient is turned on his side. The assistant holding the chest wall secures the arms, which should be straight. At this point a third assistant puts the pillows or sandbags for chest and abdomen into their correct positions. (iii) The patient is then gently rolled on to the face. The anaesthetist controls the head and neck throughout. The assistant responsible for the chest should ensure that the lower arm (the underneath arm) does not get left behind by gently drawing it towards himself as the turn on to the face takes place.

Position of the arms in the prone position. If the anaesthetist does not require access to the patient's arms, they can lie straight alongside the trunk. Alternatively, they lie on each side of the head with the arms abducted and the elbows flexed. An arm support under the mattress diagonally to the corner at the top of the table prevents them falling off. Sufficient padding should be available to protect the ulnar and radial nerves, which are particularly liable to injury. For this reason the position with arms alongside the trunk is preferable.

Turning from the prone to the supine position

It is not uncommon to turn the patient back to the supine position during the surgical procedure (for example in operations for varicose veins). The procedure for turning does not differ materially from that already described. The patient is drawn over to one side of the table and then rolled, first on to the side and then on to the back. An assistant should remove the pillows.

11 THE RECOVERY ROOM—I

At the end of the operation, instead of being taken straight back to the ward, patients remain under observation in a part of the operating suite known as the Recovery Room until the effects of the anaesthetic have passed off, and the risk of the immediate complications of the operation, i.e. reactionary haemorrhage and shock, is judged to have passed.

Continuous observation during recovery has many advantages. Complications can be dealt with as they arise by experienced staff whilst all equipment needed for resuscitation is close at hand. The occupants of the surgical wards need no longer endure the disturbance and mental stress of witnessing recovery from an operation which they themselves may undergo on the following day, whilst nursing staff no longer spend valuable time at the bedside of recovering patients at the expense of other equally pressing duties. As, however, student nurses in the wards will not obtain experience of caring for unconscious patients, arrangements should be made for them to spend some time in the recovery room where they can obtain the necessary instruction.

PLANNING AND ORGANISATION

Considerable thought has been given to the best way of siting, planning, equipping and organising a recovery room. Particular attention has been given to minimising unnecessary movement of nursing staff and keeping floor space free for transport of patients.

Siting of the Recovery Room. The Recovery Room should be between the sterile and unsterile sections of the operating suite with entry from either side. This allows ready access for medical and nursing staff in emergency and simplifies the return of the patient to the ward. Should need arise to bring patient's relatives or a minister of religion into the Recovery Room, this can be done with the minimum of disturbance.

Planning of the Recovery Room. The size and capacity of the Recovery Room depends on the number of operating theatres it serves. Two bed spaces per theatre is reasonable, but there must, in addition, be room for storage, preparation and administration. There are no partitions so that observation of patients is possible from all parts of the room. Functionally, however, the room is divided into 'areas' for patient observation (85%); for preparation and disposal (10%) (utility area); and for administration (5%). One part of the recovery area should be fitted with curtains or a cubicle for segregation of infective patients or those who are not expected to recover.

Equipment of the Recovery Room

The patient area. Each bed space is provided with piped oxygen and suction outlets, two or three electric power points, an adjustable light, and a sphygmomanometer, all attached to the wall or to a ceiling pendant. Shelving round the walls for bowls, dressings, suction catheters and patient's notes renders bedside lockers unnecessary. *Mobile shelving* (Fig. 47) large enough to hold all supplies (dressings, intravenous fluids, syringes, needles, giving sets, bowls and suction catheters) which nurses ordinarily would fetch from the utility area is a good substitute for shelves and does not interfere with observation, and being easily moved it does not obstruct movement of patients.

The patient is nursed on a 'recovery trolley' with collapsible sides which can be raised to contain a restless patient; a mechanism for tipping head up or foot down; and sockets for a drip-stand at either end.

There should be a few chairs or stools for nursing staff. Standing at the head of the patient, holding up the chin, can become very tiring on wrists and elbow joints for the nurse who is either above or below average height.

The utility area. A part of the Recovery Room designated for storage and preparation is known as the 'Utility Area'. It is fitted with cupboards, and drawers for storage with work-tops and a sink. It should contain:

1. Equipment for treatment of acute cardiac arrest (p. 154).
2. A tracheostomy set (p. 139).
3. Disposable intravenous giving sets and intravenous infusions; dextran and plasma (p. 79).
4. Drugs for (*a*) treatment of cardiac or respiratory depression

(p. 155), (*b*) reversal of muscle relaxants (p. 8), and (*c*) relief of pain.
5. Disposable syringes and hypodermic needles.
6. Suction catheters and dressings.
7. Blankets and linen.
8. Ventilators (p. 134) and monitoring equipment (p. 85).

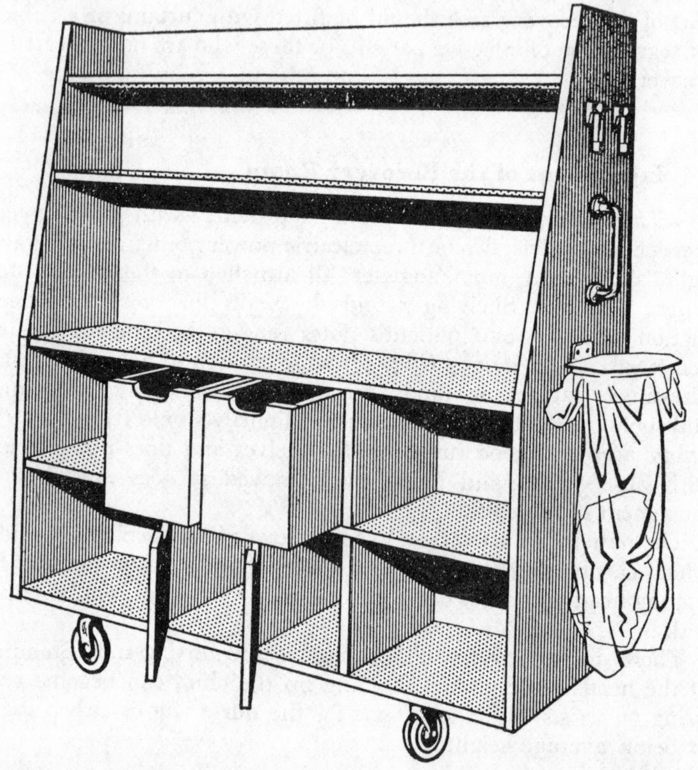

Fig. 47 Mobile shelving for recovery rooms or intensive care units

A sluice room leading off the utility area should contain a bedpan washer and steriliser, together with paper sacks for disposable equipment and containers for used equipment which has to be returned to C.S.S.D.

The administrative area. The administrative area consists simply of a desk, chair and telephone placed in a position from which it is possible to see all the patients. Although the Recovery Room is the responsibility of the Theatre Superintendent, the daily administration should be delegated to the Recovery Room Sister.

NURSING PROCEDURES

The progress of the patient through the Recovery Room consists of three phases: 1. Reception and positioning. 2. Observation. 3. Return to the ward.

Reception and Positioning

Reception. The patient arrives in the Recovery Room in charge of a member of the theatre staff who should bring a written record of the operation, the anaesthetic, and instructions for immediate post-operative care. The records should include: (i) *Patient's name*, hospital number and ward. (ii) The *nature of the operation*, details of any *drainage tubes* or *catheters* and whether suction is needed. (iii) The *anaesthetic technique* and its duration. (iv) *Estimated blood loss* and quantity and type of *intravenous fluids* given during the operation with instructions for maintenance. (v) The *condition of the patient* at the end of the operation including systolic blood pressure, pulse and respiration rates. (vi) Any *special instructions*.

Ideally the anaesthetic record should include all this information; otherwise a separate form is needed because there is always some delay before the written record of the operation becomes available to recovery room staff.

Positioning of the recovery trolley. The recovery trolley should be placed so that there is *unimpeded access to the head* because (*a*) the greater part of the nurses' attention is directed towards maintenance of a clear airway, (*b*) nine-tenths of emergencies arising during recovery concern the mouth and air passages, and (*c*) the best position to hold forward the jaw to maintain a clear airway is immediately behind the patient's head.

The head may be *towards the centre* of the room; a position which, besides giving good access, makes observation of other parts of the room easier. When the oxygen and suction outlets come from the wall, if the head is towards the centre lengths of tubing interfere with movement. In this case the head should be towards the wall, but separated by a space of not less than three feet.

The position of the patient. The '*lateral*' (or '*tonsil*') position should always be adopted unless there are good reasons to the contrary. The patient should be turned on to the side with the underarm placed *behind* the back with a pillow in front of the chest to prevent the body falling into the prone position, so that the head is low and the tongue and jaw fall forwards, clearing the airway, whilst blood, mucus or vomit can run out through the mouth.

Although this position is safest for the patient, it is not always used (i) because not all theatre or recovery trolleys are fitted with collapsible sides to retain bulky or restless patients who, in the lateral position might fall off the trolley during the journey from theatre to recovery room, and (ii) the nature of the operation makes it impracticable for example after (a) *orthopaedic* operations: when the patient is in plaster and the position may be impossible, (b) *chest* operations: lying on the unoperated side may embarrass respiration

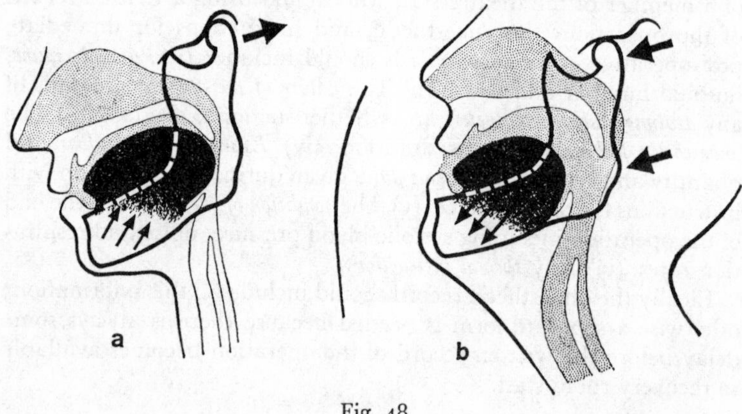

Fig. 48

a Obstructed respiration by the tongue in the supine position
b Clearance by airway and lifting the jaw forward

whilst lying on the operated side could cause harm especially when ribs have been resected, (c) *plastic* operations: when skin grafting procedures have been undertaken and adoption of the lateral position may be unwise for fear of disturbing the grafted areas or a pedicle graft and (*d*) after certain ophthalmic operations.

When the patient remains on the back, danger of obstruction to respiration by the tongue falling into the back of the throat is constantly present. It can best be kept clear by inserting an oral airway (Fig. 48), turning the head to one side and sliding the jaw forwards. An oral airway should not confer a false sense of security as respiration can still become obstructed. If necessary the jaw should be held forward until control of the airway has returned (see below).

Observation of the patient. When the patient is in position breathing freely with an unobstructed airway, attention should be given to the following:

(*a*) *The wound dressing* should be secure and dry. If soaked in blood, it will require packing with application of firmer pressure. If this is ineffective, the surgeon should be informed.

(*b*) *Drainage tubes*, if present, should be secure. *Chest drainage* tubes should be attached to an *under-water seal. Large skin wounds* (for example, radical amputation of the breast) often have vacuum suction ('Redivac') bottles attached. *Blood loss* should not exceed 25–50 ml, but after some orthopaedic operations greater loss can be expected.

(*c*) *After operations on an arm or leg, or application of a plaster cast, limbs should be left uncovered and open to view*, and regularly inspected for adequacy of the circulation i.e. fingers or toes should be pink and warm.

(*d*) *Intravenous infusions* should be secured (using if necessary a lightly padded splint), and adjusted to flow at the prescribed rate. If flow stops or fluid runs into the tissues it should be reported immediately.

(*e*) *Naso-gastric (Ryle's) tubes* should be made secure with adhesive tape. A spigot, if present, should be removed and replaced by a small plastic bag. Aspiration should be performed as ordered and aspirate labelled and retained for inspection. *Bladder catheters* (usual after gynaecological and urological operations and abdomino-perineal resection) should be secured and attached to a sterile urine bag or bottle.

(*f*) *Pulse, respiration and blood pressure* should be recorded every 15 minutes until consciousness returns. Regular observations of these signs help early recognition of the onset of post-operative shock, reactionary haemorrhage or respiratory depression.

(*g*) *Oxygen* should be given by mask or nasal catheter. Although there may be no obvious signs of oxygen lack some degree of reduced oxygen in the blood (hypoxaemia) occurs after every operation.

Progress of normal recovery. Normal recovery following general anaesthesia can be said to occur if there is (*a*) a progressive return of consciousness, (*b*) the pulse and respiration rates remain within normal limits and (*c*) there is a steady return of systolic blood pressure towards the pre-operative figure.

The return to consciousness becomes evident from the re-appearance of reflex activity which always takes place in the reverse order to its disappearance during induction. The journey from relatively deep anaesthesia to awareness is marked by the consecutive appearance of groups of reflexes each of which could be called milestones on the road to recovery. The significant reflexes in the order of their return are: (i) *Tracheal, laryngeal* and *cough* reflexes. (ii) *Reflex activity* of the small muscles of the jaw and eye. (iii) *Swallowing and vomiting* reflexes. (iv) *Response to painful stimuli.* (v) *Response to the spoken word.*

(i) *The tracheal, laryngeal and cough reflexes* which protect the respiratory tract recover first. Their presence is evident if gentle movement or deflation of the cuff of the endotracheal tube induces straining and breath holding. As a rule this stage has been reached and the tube removed before arrival in the recovery room, but there are occasions when the tube is left in position in order to protect the airway (*a*) after operations on the nose or in the mouth (including dental extractions), or where splints have been applied to the jaw (*b*) following removal of large tumours of the thyroid gland (which may have displaced the trachea or weakened the tracheal cartilages by pressure); and (*c*) in the presence of inflammatory swellings in the neck (a cause of oedema and obstruction of the larynx).

The tube is also left in position when respiration is inadequate after operation. It should remain until the presence of swallowing movements (see below) indicates that return of consciousness is imminent, and should not be removed until ordered. When permission is given, the patient should be turned on the side, an oral airway inserted and the tube withdrawn after careful aspiration of secretions from the pharynx.

(ii) *Return of reflex muscular movement.* As depth of anaesthesia decreases there is a general return of reflex muscular activity, beginning with the larger muscles, and progressing until activity of the smaller muscles, particularly of the tongue, the jaw, and the eyeball indicate that full recovery is not far removed. At this stage, (*a*) an oral airway induces contraction of the masseter muscle of the jaw and attempts to open the mouth will be resisted. (*b*) On *raising the eyelids*, slow eccentric movements of the eyeball can be seen (a sign sometimes known as the 'roving eyeball'), whilst (*c*) movements of muscles on either side of the lower jaw indicate the imminent return of swallowing and vomiting reflexes.

Caution. The conjunctival and corneal reflexes (reflex closure of the eyelid following a light touch with the fingertip to the conjunctiva or cornea) do not provide any information which cannot be obtained in other ways and may introduce infection or damage the cornea.

(iii) *The return of swallowing and vomiting reflexes* is accompanied by a change from automatic respiration to interrupted breathing of varying depth because respiration is inhibited during swallowing. *A patient who can swallow can also vomit*; so this stage requires close attention. Since respiration also ceases during vomiting, a change to quiet shallow breathing which suddenly stops, can be a sign of impending vomiting. With return of swallowing and vomiting reflexes, contact of the tip of the airway with the back of the throat can provoke retching which may be averted by withdrawing the airway an inch or two. This should not lead to obstructed breathing because return of muscle tone prevents the tongue falling backwards. The airway will eventually be rejected by the patient.

(iv) *Motor response to painful stimuli.* Soon after return of swallowing reflexes, painful stimuli, e.g. squeezing the lobe of the ear, or firm pressure on the sternum will induce movement of limbs or contraction of the orbital muscles round the eye.

(v) *Response to the spoken word.* Recovery of consciousness is complete when response can be obtained to the spoken word shown by opening of the eyes and efforts to speak.

Relief of pain during recovery. The need for pain relief during recovery depends on (*a*) whether opiates have been included in the pre-operative medication, or in the technique of anaesthesia, and (*b*) the nature of the surgery.

Patients who have not received opiates pre-operatively complain of pain sooner than those who have, and if intravenous opiates have been given as part of the anaesthetic technique, the need for pain relief on recovery may be delayed for some hours. Severe pain may follow operations on bones and joints and such patients often need early relief of pain. Post-operative instructions should therefore always include a prescription for an analgesic injection, otherwise delay may occur and the patient suffer unnecessarily.

Sometimes the injection of an opiate causes a sharp fall in blood pressure. Pain impulses stimulate activity of the sympathetic nervous system raising blood pressure. Sudden pain relief reduces sympathetic activity so that blood pressure may fall. Opiates also induce depression of respiration. Patients should not therefore be returned to the ward until *half an hour after an injection* of an opiate for pain relief when any effects on blood pressure or respiration will have become evident.

Return to the Ward

Recovery should be complete within half to one hour of arrival in the recovery room. The patient is ready to return to the ward if: (*a*) *consciousness has returned* shown by response to pain and the spoken word. (*b*) *Blood pressure, pulse and respiration rates* are stable indicating absence of complications (see below). (*c*) *The wound dressing is dry, drainage tubes are in place*, and suction operating correctly.

Checking of the patient before return to the ward. In some hospitals, patient's condition is checked by an anaesthetist before leaving the recovery room; elsewhere this is left to the Sister in Charge, who only calls for medical advice if there are instructions to do so or if complications make it necessary. Whoever takes the patient to the ward should be given *full details of the patient's progress, together with instructions for further care, in writing.* Maintenance of the chain of communication—theatre—recovery room—ward is essential for intelligent care by nursing staff.

Recovery following Local or Regional Anaesthesia

Patients who have undergone operations with subdural, epidural or regional nerve blocks (Chapter 20) may not be fully conscious on arrival in the recovery room because it is becoming a common practice to induce a mild state of unconsciousness with intravenous agents such as diazepan (Valium) or pethidine and promethazine. Attention to the airway may therefore be necessary until the reappearance of swallowing reflexes indicates return of control.

All patients should remain under observation until the effects of the local anaesthetic have worn off completely and the stability of the circulatory system indicates the absence of reactionary haemorrhage or shock.

The effects of the local anaesthetic can be said to have worn off when full sensation has returned to the area involved and, if subdural or epidural methods have been used, full muscular power has returned.

Tests should be made to ensure the presence of sensation to heat, cold, and pain stimuli (by gentle pin prick). Return of muscular power can be assessed by ability to move the lower limbs.

After subdural or epidural block there is always some fall in blood pressure which may often be below pre-operative level on arrival in the recovery room. It is temporarily intensified by movement involved in transfer from operating table to recovery trolley. The patient should be kept flat and the foot of the bed raised for a short period until systolic pressure begins to rise.

Note. Too frequent blood pressure estimations disturb a conscious patient and should be avoided unless there are specific indications for repeated observations.

Pain will require relief by injection of opiates as the local anaesthetic wears off.

12 THE RECOVERY ROOM—II

Complications of recovery can be attributed either to the *anaesthetic*, or the *operation*.

ANAESTHETIC COMPLICATIONS

Anaesthetic complications arise from (1) *respiratory obstruction* or (2) *respiratory depression*.

(1) Respiratory obstruction. Respiratory obstruction should *not* occur if the patient is nursed in the lateral position (p. 107), with the head low and the mouth below the level of the laryngeal opening. Obstruction may be *anatomical* (from the tongue) or *reflex* (from laryngeal closure).

Anatomical obstruction happens if the tongue falls back against the pharyngeal wall, occluding the pharynx so that air cannot enter the lungs (Fig. 48a). It may be *complete* or *partial*. *Complete obstruction* is noiseless, but evident from *retraction of the chest muscles* (in an attempt to fill the lungs), and from cyanosis (blueness) of the skin; a sign which can easily be missed in patients with pigmented skins. *Partial obstruction* is always noisy. Audible breathing indicates partial obstruction with certainty.

Treatment. (i) The obstruction can be relieved by sliding the lower jaw forward carrying the tongue with it and thus clearing the airway and allowing the insertion of an oral airway of a suitable size (p. 53). If these measures fail to relieve obstruction search should be made for foreign material in the pharynx, e.g. dental packs or gauze swabs.

To draw the jaw forwards place both hands behind the ascending ramus of the jaw and lift it forward by sliding it along the supra-condylar notch in the upper jaw (Fig. 48b). Holding the point of the chin will not maintain a clear airway. If an airway is already in place (*and an airway is no guarantee against obstruction*), it should be removed, replaced correctly or substituted by a larger one. (ii)

Unless there are contra-indications (p. 108), the patient should be turned on to the side. (iii) If obstruction has been severe, oxygen should be given.

Reflex obstruction from laryngeal spasm occurs when closure of the vocal cords occurs following contact with mucus, blood or vomited material. *When complete*, the signs are those of oxygen lack: congestion and cyanosis of the head and neck with retraction of the chest and contraction of the accessory muscles of respiration (alae nasi and sterno-mastoid). *Incomplete or partial obstruction* is more common and is audible as respiratory stridor, or 'crowning' respiration.

Treatment. Complete laryngeal obstruction is a major emergency which can lead to cardiac arrest and requires rapid and energetic treatment. Oxygen should be given liberally and medical assistance summoned, meanwhile (*a*) the patient is turned on to the *lateral position* with the head lower than the chest, to ensure that blood or vomitus will run out of the mouth, thus preventing inhalation should the vocal cords relax. (*b*) Secretions in the pharynx should be aspirated by passing a suction catheter through the nose, whilst attempts are made to open the clenched jaws with the help of a wooden wedge (p. 57) and the insertion of a Mason-Ferguson gag (p. 58).

Partial laryngeal obstruction should be treated in the same way as total obstruction: administration of oxygen, adoption of the lateral position and pharyngeal aspiration.

(2) Respiratory Depression

Depressed respiration during recovery may be *central* or *peripheral* in origin.

(i) *Central depression* arises from the effects of opiates and anaesthetics on the central nervous mechanisms controlling respiration (p. 121). Respiration is of inadequate *depth* and *rate* (below 10 per minute). Cyanosis (a bluish tinge of the lips) may be present but is obscured by administration of oxygen and difficult to detect in subjects with pigmented skins. *Treatment* is by administration of oxygen pending intravenous injection of *morphine antagonists* (p. 187) if opiates are the cause; or of *respiratory stimulants* (p. 190), which will restore normal breathing.

(ii) *Peripheral depression* is due to muscular weakness following administration of muscle relaxants and is not infrequently associated with some degree of circulatory depression. It can be distinguished from central depression because (*a*) the *rate* of respiration is normal or increased, (*b*) a 'tracheal tug' is often present which is seen as forceful depression of the trachea and thyroid cartilage with each inspiratory effort. As the intercostal muscles cannot expand the chest, when the diaphragm contracts it pulls the lungs downwards and (*c*) normal respiratory rhythm is reversed, a pause occurring *after inspiration* instead of expiration, giving respiration a 'gasping' character. *Treatment.* Oxygen should be administered, an anaesthetist summoned, and the following prepared (*a*) laryngoscope and endotracheal tube for re-intubation if the tube has already been removed; (*b*) a ventilator; and (*c*) neostigmin and atropine for reversal of curare and similar relaxants (p. 8).

COMPLICATIONS ARISING FROM THE OPERATION

Complications of surgery during recovery are *haemorrhage* and *shock.* Haemorrhage, reactionary in nature, may occur *externally* or *internally*.

Haemorrhage

(i) *External haemorrhage* will be evident since the wound dressing will be soaked in blood. Haemorrhage from a tooth socket or following tonsillectomy may not be immediately obvious because the blood is swallowed, only becoming apparent after vomiting. This may occur particularly after dental extractions; tonsillectomy; or plastic surgery for a cleft palate.

(ii) *Internal haemorrhage* presents a similar picture to post-operative shock and the signs—rapid pulse, falling blood-pressure, pallor and sweating are the same.

Post-operative shock. During recovery shock may arise from (i) *Reactionary haemorrhage* (see above), (ii) the combined effects of *haemorrhage and operative trauma*, (iii) *bacterial toxins*; i.e. peritoneal infection from appendicitis or perforation of the bowel; or following surgery of the bladder and prostate where secondary infection is common. The bacteria are of the 'gram negative' variety and the toxins they produce are released following their destruction by the defensive mechanisms of the body, or by antibiotics and this variety of shock is known as 'gram negative' shock.

The signs of shock arise from failure of perfusion, due to vasoconstriction, which, initially protective in purpose, gives rise to oxygen lack, and if continued unchecked causes capillary paralysis and dilation. Blood accumulates in the capillaries (whose capacity is enormous) and its return to the heart is prevented by constriction of the veins. The volume of circulating blood falls progressively and becomes inadequate to provide sufficient oxygen for vital organs like the liver, the kidney and the intestines, so that in the absence of energetic resuscitation, a condition known as 'irreversible shock' supervenes which resists all forms of treatment.

Whatever the cause, the early signs (during which the condition responds to treatment) and can be diagnosed from the appearance of the patient, associated with characteristic changes in the *rate* and *character* of the pulse and in the blood pressure.

(*a*) *The appearance of the patient.* Sweating and pallor of the skin, a blue tinge of the lips and finger-nails and coldness of the tip of the nose to the back of the hand.

(*b*) *Changes in pulse and blood-pressure.* The pulse becomes 'thready' (i.e. difficult to feel because the artery is constricted) and the *rate* increases. The systolic blood-pressure, though it may be maintained in the early stages, ultimately begins to fall.

The *appearance* of the patient is of greater significance than change in the blood-pressure. The presence of sweating, pallor, blue finger-nails and a nose that is cold to the back of the hand are sufficient reason to call for medical assistance (the surgeon or anaesthetist) and to adopt the treatment for shock.

Treatment. Treatment of shock is aimed at overcoming oxygen lack and restoring the peripheral circulation by: (i) administration of oxygen by nasal catheter or mask should begin immediately; (ii) opening the intravenous infusion to its fullest extent, and if flow is not rapid, recourse should be had to the hand pump. If blood is not running, it should be prepared for immediate infusion. If blood is not available, a plasma expander (Dextran) may be substituted. Intravenous fluids increase the volume of circulating fluid, and by increasing output of the heart improve perfusion and oxygenation. (iii) The foot of the bed should be raised to encourage return of blood to the heart and improve flow to the brain.

Clinical improvement is seen from (*a*) decrease of vaso-constriction with restoration of peripheral perfusion so that the skin becomes warm and dry with pink nail beds, and (*b*) improvement of pulse volume, a fall in pulse rate, and a rise in the systolic blood-pressure.

Shock following Subdural or Epidural Anaesthesia

Subdural and epidural anaesthesia have a reputation for reducing the severity of operative shock, in part, but not wholly explained by the dry operative fields obtained with these methods so that blood loss is less than under general anaesthesia. In some instances signs of shock may appear as the effects of the anaesthetic wear off. After operations on the prostate, for which these methods are popular, vaso-constriction and shivering may occur during recovery and the patient complains of feeling cold. These signs indicate the presence of some degree of 'gram negative' shock and arise from disturbance of tissues already infected with gram negative bacteria and release of their endotoxins into the general circulation.

Treatment should be (*a*) to keep the patient warm, (*b*) speed up the intravenous infusion (*c*) and inform the doctor in charge. Rapid improvement may follow intravenous injection of twenty-five milli-grammes of chlorpromazine.

Drugs in the Treatment of Shock

In addition to the above measures, drugs may be used to overcome shock. There are (i) vasopressors; (ii) vasodilators; (iii) steroids (hydrocortisone).

(i) *Vasopressors* (p. 191). Vasopressors are administered in the treatment of shock *in addition to I.V. fluids and oxygen*, to increase the force of contraction of the heart and *raise* the systolic blood-pressure in an attempt to improve the flow of blood to the periphery. *Isoprenaline* ('Isuprel') is used for this purpose because besides increasing the force of contraction of the heart it dilates the blood vessels of the muscles.

(ii) *Vasodilators. Chlorpromazine* ('Largactil') or *phenoxybenzamine* ('Dibenzyline') have been advocated for *prevention* or *treatment* of shock for their vasodilator effects which open up the blood vessels, improve perfusion and restore peripheral circulation. Vasodilation increases the capacity of the blood vessels and may cause further fall in blood-pressure unless accompanied by liberal infusion of fluids when blood-pressure rises.

Chlorpromazine (or 'Largactil') may also be given during anaesthesia to prevent development of shock. During recovery systolic pressure may be lower than normal, but if perfusion remains adequate, as evidenced by dry warm skin and pink finger-nails, this low figure need not give rise to anxiety, and there will be a progressive rise during recovery. If this does not occur, the presence of reactionary haemorrhage should be suspected, because apart from pallor, the signs of shock from haemorrhage—vaso-constriction, sweating, etc. may not be apparent.

(iii) *Steroids* (*hydrocortisone*). Large doses of hydrocortisone have been shown to prevent development of experimental shock, especially that arising from infection of the peritoneum ('Gram negative' shock, peritonitis). They produce a mild state of vasodilation and are less likely to cause a fall in blood-pressure than vasodilator drugs.

13 RESPIRATORY FAILURE—I: The Physiology of Normal Respiration

A brief revision of the physiology of *normal* respiration should precede discussion of the causes of *failure* in order to understand why respiratory failure occurs and the measures taken to treat it.

The purpose of respiration is to provide enough oxygen to meet the needs of living cells and to remove the carbon dioxide they produce. It is maintained through three interdependent processes: *Ventilation*, *Diffusion*, and *Perfusion* (Fig. 49).

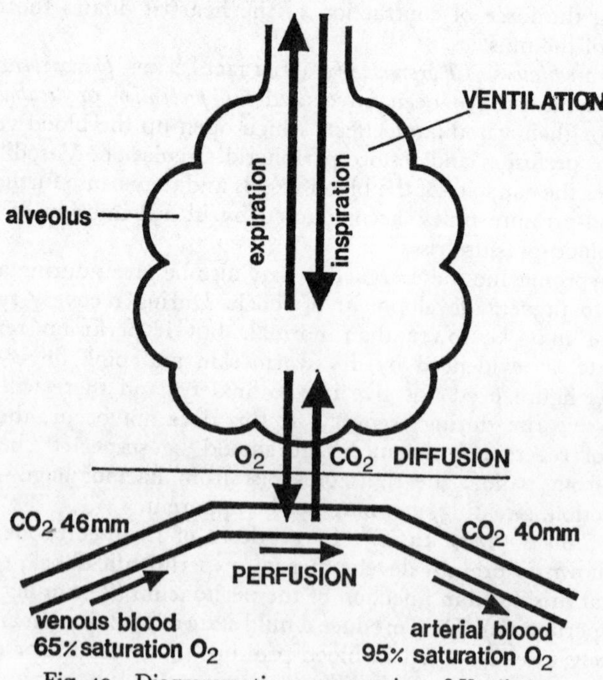

Fig. 49 Diagrammatic representation of *Ventilation*, *Diffusion* and *Perfusion*

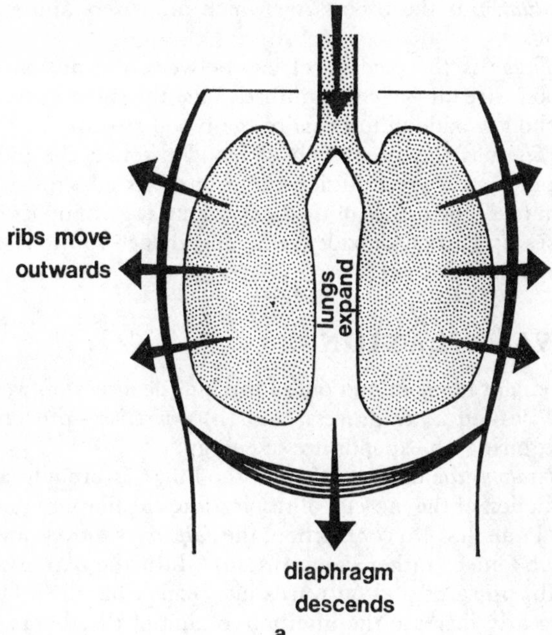

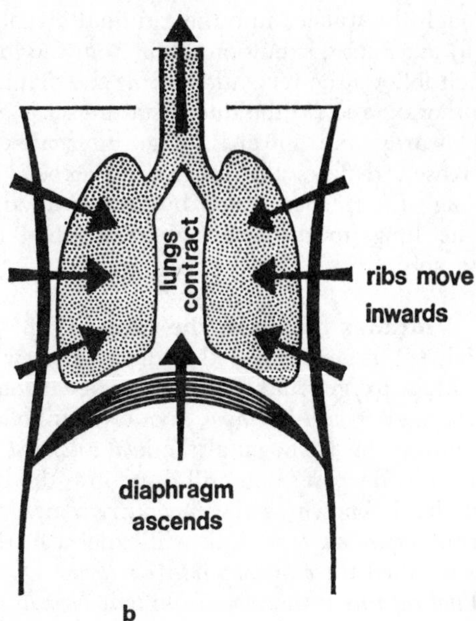

Fig. 50 Mechanics of respiration

a inspiration b expiration

(1) *Ventilation* is the process by which air enters and leaves the lungs.

(2) *Diffusion* is the passage of gas between the alveoli and the blood stream—oxygen diffuses *into* the blood stream and carbon dioxide diffuses *out* of the blood stream.

(3) *Perfusion* is the circulation of blood through the pulmonary capillaries where diffusion occurs, and its subsequent circulation to all the tissues of the body where it gives up oxygen and takes up carbon dioxide, returning thence to the right heart and lungs.

1. VENTILATION

The movement of air in and out of the lungs consists of two phases: (i) *inspiration*—an *active* process, and (ii) *expiration*—predominantly *passive*, requiring no expenditure of energy.

(i) *Inspiration*, the entry of air into the lungs, is brought about by the contraction of the muscles of respiration, the diaphragm and the intercostal muscles. On contraction, the *diaphragm* moves downwards into the abdomen (rather like a piston) whilst the *intercostal muscles* lift the ribs upwards and outwards like bucket handles. These two actions greatly increase the internal volume of the thorax and the lungs expand to fill the empty space created, drawing air down through the trachea into the terminal alveoli (Fig. 50a).

(ii) *Expiration*, expulsion of air from the lungs, is a *passive* process which follows the relaxation of (*a*) the diaphragm, which rises into the thorax, and (*b*) the intercostal muscles, allowing the ribs to fall downwards and inwards. The internal volume of the thorax decreases, deflates the lungs, and expels the contained air out through the trachea, aided by the contraction of the elastic fibres of the lungs to their normal unstretched length ('elastic recoil') (Fig. 50b).

Volumes of air in the lungs (Fig. 51). The volume of air [illegible]ich enters and leaves the lungs varies with the demand of the [illegible]es for oxygen and the quantity of carbon dioxide they produce. [illegible] *normal quiet breathing*, about 500 ml of air passes in and out of [illegible]s; this is known as the *tidal volume*. Continuation of inspira- [illegible] deepest point will draw into the lungs a further 1500 ml [illegible] known as the *inspiratory reserve volume*. Continuation of [illegible]*tion to its limit* will expel a further 1500 ml of air and [illegible]e *expiratory reserve volume*.

[illegible] the *sum* of the *three preceding volumes* and represents [illegible] from *maximal expiration to maximal inspiration*, [illegible]erage figure of 3½ litres (3500 ml).

Dead space air. During quiet expiration, one third of the air expired (150 ml) remains in the upper air passages. This is known as 'dead space air'. At the next inspiration it mixes with the fresh air entering the lungs, raising the carbon dioxide content and reducing available oxygen. Dead space is of no significance in *normal* subjects. Increase of dead space with accumulation of carbon dioxide occurs in some anaesthetic circuits, especially when breathing is depressed or (as in children) tidal volume is low.

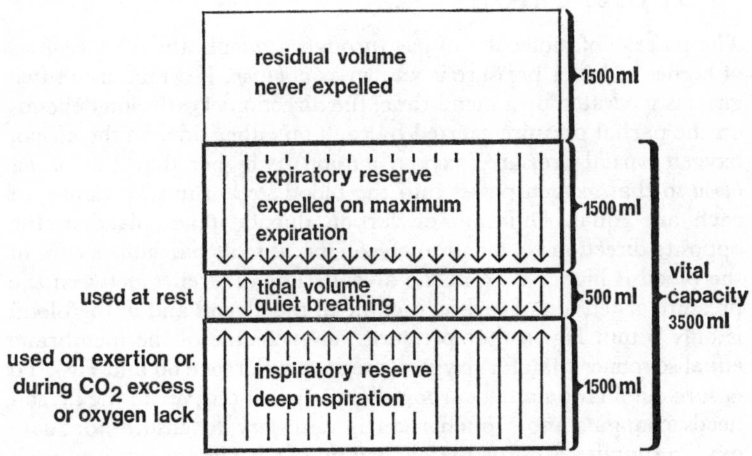

Fig. 51 Schematic representation of volume of air in lungs

Control of ventilation. The rate and depth of breathing is controlled by the *respiratory centre* in the lower part of the brain stem (medulla oblongata). It consists of a diffuse collection of nerve cells which regulate the rate and depth of ventilation through the phrenic and intercostal nerves which supply the diaphragm and intercostal muscles. Its regulatory effect on respiration is determined by a constant flow of information from (*a*) other parts of the brain (fear and emotion can cause rapid breathing); (*b*) from peripheral sensory nerves (pain and cold can stimulate breathing); (*c*) from sensory fibres of the vagus and glossopharyngeal nerves in the trachea, larynx, and pharynx whose stimulation can *inhibit* breathing, for example during vomiting; (*d*) from specialised collections of nerve fibres in the lungs, 'stretch receptors', which record the degree of inflation or deflation; (*e*) from nerve receptors in the carotid arteries and the aorta which convey information about the oxyg content in the circulating blood.

Chemical control. The degree of acidity and carbon dioxide content of the blood also influence breathing through the respiratory centre which is exquisitely sensitive to carbon dioxide. The smallest rise in blood content instantly increases the rate and depth of respiration. Lowering of the carbon dioxide content of the blood by voluntary overbreathing or by hyperventilation during anaesthesia, depresses respiration, which ceases until the blood level of carbon dioxide returns once more to normal.

2. DIFFUSION

The passage of molecules of gas through a membrane from regions of higher to lower pressure is known as *diffusion*. If a mixture of two gases is separated by a membrane, the direction of diffusion depends on the partial pressure exerted by each on either side. In the *alveoli*, oxygen partial pressure (oxygen tension) is higher than that *in the blood* so that oxygen passes into the blood stream until pressures of each are equal. Diffusion of carbon dioxide takes place in the opposite direction i.e. blood to alveoli, because its partial pressure in the blood is higher than in the alveoli. The difference between the pressure or tension of carbon dioxide in the alveoli and in the blood is only 6 mm Hg so that pressures on each side of the membrane equalise sooner than for oxygen (pressure difference 60 mm Hg). To ensure elimination of all carbon dioxide produced, air in the alveoli needs changing more often than is necessary to ensure adequate oxygen supplies. Approximately 250 ml of oxygen are required each minute at rest, and 250 ml of carbon dioxide need elimination. Each *100 ml of expired air carries away 5 ml of carbon dioxide*, so to remove 250 ml, *5 litres (5,000 ml) of air must be breathed each minute*, although 250 ml of oxygen could be obtained from a much smaller quantity. For this reason, elimination of carbon dioxide presents greater problems than oxygenation in treatment of respiratory failure, and under certain conditions (p. 127) oxygen therapy can do more harm han good. Also, for this reason the total flow of gases during aesthesia with rebreathing should exceed 5 litres per minute to re adequate elimination of carbon dioxide.

ERFUSION

the vascular element of respiration. In order that ve) can take place, blood must be transported to the ary membrane and, after oxygenation it must be eft side of the heart, from whence it is driven to the ic peripheral circulation to perfuse all the tissues

The pumping action of the heart is responsible for the maintenance of perfusion, but to do this efficiently it must receive adequate quantities of venous blood from the tissues and of oxygenated blood from the lungs and at the same time the heart muscle must be adequately perfused with oxygenated blood via the coronary arteries.

14 RESPIRATORY FAILURE—II: The Causes and Principles of Treatment

RESPIRATORY FAILURE

Respiratory failure occurs when (*a*) it is no longer possible to maintain sufficient oxygen in the blood stream to meet the body's needs or (*b*) elimination of the carbon dioxide resulting from cellular metabolism is inadequate so that the amount in the blood accumulates progressively above normal limits. *The onset may be rapid*, when all its manifestations, being those of sudden death, will be obvious; or, it may be insidious and only detected by estimations of the amount of oxygen and carbon dioxide in the blood stream. There are many causes, all of which can be attributed to a disorder of one or more of the components of normal respiration, *Ventilation*, *Diffusion* and *Perfusion* (Chapter 14).

Respiratory Failure from Disorders of Ventilation

Failure of ventilation arises from (*a*) *inadequate muscular activity*, (*b*) *damage*, *infection* or *poisoning* of the *respiratory centres in the brain*, and (*c*) *damage to the rib cage* following injury.

(*a*) *Muscular failure* occurs in the course of *acute poliomyelitis* when amage of the nerve cells in the spinal cord responsible for muscular vity causes widespread paralysis which may involve the muscles piration. A less common cause is hereditary wasting of muscles, as '*muscular dystrophy*'. Progressive wasting of all voluntary occurs to an extent that, although able to maintain ventilast, the extra-ventilatory effort which acute pulmonary y demand leads to respiratory failure.

to the respiratory centres may follow intracranial haemorncephalitis; or poisoning by drugs (particularly rates).

rib cage from multiple rib fractures after road y the rigidity of the thoracic cage and may

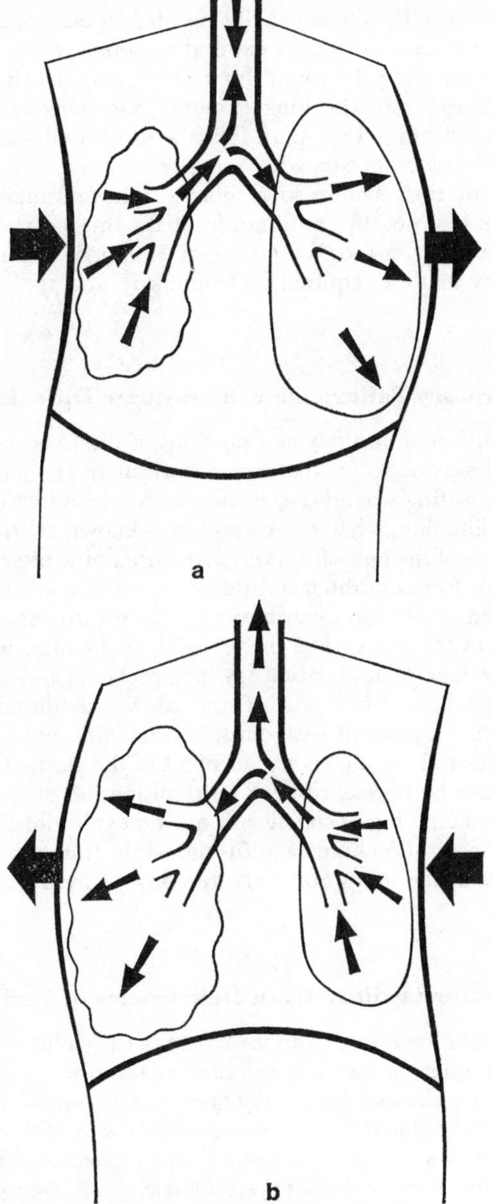

Fig. 52 Paradoxical respiration from 'Flail In' chest

a *Inspiration* Damaged side moves inwards, stale air expressed and vitia fresh gases entering sound side

b *Expiration* Damaged side expands and draws stale air from sound s

give rise to a disorder of ventilation known as '*paradoxical respiration*'. During *inspiration*, the damaged ribs are drawn *inwards* compressing the underlying lung so that its expired air mixes with, and dilutes the fresh air entering the sound lung (Fig. 52a). During *expiration*, the *ribs move outwards*, the lung expands but *draws in* expired air from the sound lung (Fig. 52b). Thus a rapid build-up of carbon dioxide in the blood occurs with progressive reduction of available oxygen. Respiratory failure soon follows unless normal respiratory movement is restored by stabilisation of the injured chest wall (by sandbags or traction) or by artificial inflation of the lungs (a tracheostomy may be required) (Chapters 16 and 17).

Respiratory Failure from Inadequate Diffusion

Failure of diffusion occurs when portions of the lungs collapse and become airless, due to (*a*) the presence of air in the pleural cavity (from a perforating wound of the chest or from rupture of the lung) preventing inflation, when the condition is known as '*pneumothorax*', or (*b*) collapse of the lungs from restricted breathing after abdominal operations or from an abnormal reflex, when it is known as '*atelectasis*'. Failure of diffusion can also arise in the course of *pneumonic inflammation* of the lungs when the alveoli become filled with inflammatory secretions ('consolidation'), which prevent gaseous exchange. Respiratory failure from any of the above conditions is more likely to occur in patients with chronic bronchitis and emphysema. Chronic bronchitis results in replacement of the elastic tissue in the lung substance by fibrous tissue. The resulting loss of elasticity prevents proper emptying of the alveoli during expiration; overdistension during inspiration hinders diffusion, whilst frothy sputum in the deeper parts of the lungs obstructs free flow of fresh gases.

Respiratory Failure from Deficiencies of Perfusion

of perfusion is due to an *inadequacy* of the circulation of blood
he lungs, or loss of *oxygen carrying capacity*.
circulation follows (*a*) *failure of the pumping action of* the
rt failure from any cause with slowing of the circulation
ient oxygen reaches the cells; especially of the heart,
liver and kidneys; (*b*) *loss of circulating fluid* from
dehydration when there is insufficient blood to
tissues from the lungs. Deficient perfusion and
fied if the blood passes directly from arterioles

to venules, bypassing the alveolar capillaries, a condition known as 'shunting'.

Loss of oxygen-carrying capacity results from lack of red cells due to haemorrhage or anaemia; or from carbon monoxide poisoning when the formation of carboxyhaemoglobin renders the red blood cells incapable of taking up oxygen.

Principles of Treatment of Respiratory Failure

Although respiratory failure develops gradually and in its early stages may not be immediately recognised, its course is relentlessly progressive because the response to the rising carbon dioxide content of the blood intensifies oxygen lack and starts what may be called the 'vicious circle' of respiratory failure.

The steady increase of carbon dioxide in the blood, through its action on the respiratory centre, stimulates respiration. The added muscular effort involved in improving ventilation unfortunately *intensifies the shortage of oxygen* and *produces more carbon dioxide* creating a vicious circle in which increased respiratory effort—intensified oxygen lack—further carbon dioxide production; repeats itself, leading ultimately to death from oxygen shortage and carbon dioxide poisoning.

Treatment aims at breaking the 'vicious circle', and is directed towards (*a*) *overcoming oxygen lack* by providing additional oxygen to improve ventilation and carbon dioxide elimination, and (*b*) treatment of the underlying cause: for example, antibiotics for lung infection; digitalis for heart failure; resuscitation for shock and surgery for chest injuries. *Administration of oxygen alone* may be sufficient to overcome carbon dioxide retention (see Oxygen Therapy). If, however, oxygen is not effective, or if *carbon dioxide narcosis* (mental confusion followed by loss of consciousness) occurs, further measures are required. These are (*a*) assisted respiration by a ventilator, and subsequently (*b*) a tracheostomy.

OXYGEN THERAPY

Oxygen therapy is the treatment of oxygen lack in the tissues by adding oxygen to the inspired air. It should not be confused with 'hyperbaric' oxygen therapy (p. 131) in which patients are exposed to oxygen under high pressure.

Equipment for Oxygen Therapy

In recovery rooms and intensive care units, piped oxygen is available, but elsewhere in the hospital the source may be from cylinders.

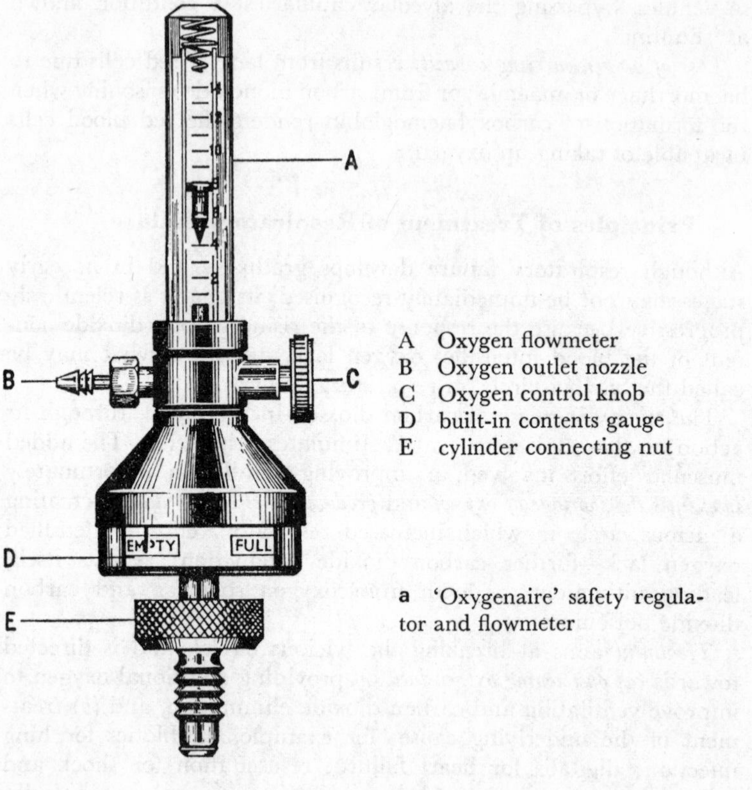

A Oxygen flowmeter
B Oxygen outlet nozzle
C Oxygen control knob
D built-in contents gauge
E cylinder connecting nut

a 'Oxygenaire' safety regulator and flowmeter

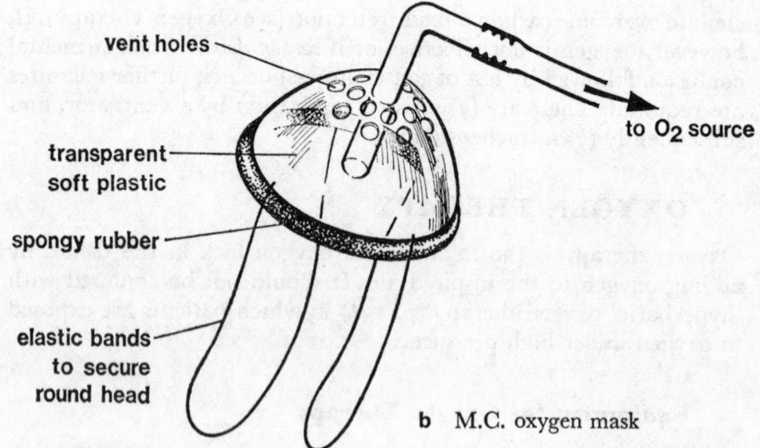

b M.C. oxygen mask

Fig. 53a and b Equipment for oxygen therapy

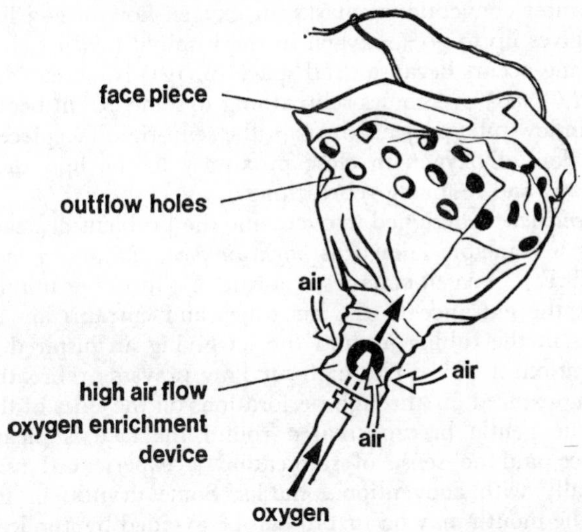

Fig. 53c Equipment for oxygen therapy

Vent face mask showing principle of high air flow with oxygen enrichment ('HAFOE')

Whenever prolonged oxygen therapy is contemplated, the patient should, if possible, be brought to a piped supply, which is cheaper, whilst no labour is involved in changing and moving heavy cylinders.

Some means of measuring the flow of gases is necessary. Piped outlets for oxygen have standard flow-meters and a control tap. Cylinders should be fitted with a flow-meter in addition to a reducing valve. The Oxygenaire Safety Regulator (Fig. 53a) is an example. It consists of a combined reducing valve, flow-meter and flow-regulator, which fits directly into the cylinder head. An outlet nozzle takes the connecting tubing for the patient. A built-in 'Contents Gauge' gives good warning when a change of cylinder may be necessary.

The source of oxygen can be brought to the patient in three ways: (i) by face mask, (ii) through a nasal catheter, and (iii) in an oxygen tent.

(i) *Face masks* for oxygen therapy resemble anaesthetic face pieces but are lighter, disposable, and can be fixed in position by means of rubber bands. The ideal mask should (*a*) fit snugly over the face giving a leak-proof seal without causing discomfort, and (*b*) be sufficiently light in weight not to fall off or become displaced by movement of the head.

With most conventional masks an oxygen flow of 2–3 litres per minute gives up to 30% oxygen in the inspired mixture, but some rebreathing occurs because dead space (p. 121) is increased.

The M.C. mask overcomes rebreathing to some extent because the oxygen inflow tube projects through the semi-rigid facepiece directing the flow of oxygen in close proximity to the lips, displacing expired air, and reducing rebreathing.

The Ventimask is designed to overcome the problem of dead space by using a principle known as '*high air flow with oxygen enrichment*' (H.A.F.O.E.). Oxygen emerges at a rate of 4 litres per minute from a jet (at the entrance to the air tube) and entrains air through apertures in the tubing around the jet giving an inspired oxygen concentration of 28%. The high air flow prevents rebreathing by displacing expired air through perforations on the sides of the facepiece. The gentle breeze created round the face is pleasant to experience and no sense of suffocation is experienced as occurs occasionally with conventional masks. Some dryness of the skin around the mouth may occur but can be avoided by application of cream or lip salve. The Ventimask is used for patients in whom carbon dioxide accumulation is likely, e.g. chronic bronchitis. The 'candlestick' shape renders it more readily displaced by movement than conventional masks.

Nasal catheters. A rubber or plastic catheter passed through the nose into the pharynx and secured to the face with adhesive tape is a simple and effective way of giving oxygen. A flow rate of 3–4 litres per minute will maintain inspired oxygen concentration at 30% without increasing dead space, and is not reduced greatly by mouth breathing. It is useful for confused or restless patients for whom a face mask involves constant adjustment. A more sophisticated method of giving nasal oxygen is by means of a modified spectacle frame which carries tubing for a catheter in each nostril.

Transparent plastic *oxygen tents* which cover a bed provide an oxygen enriched atmosphere. Although comfortable for the patient, the oxygen concentration falls whenever the tent is opened as may frequently be necessary to carry out nursing procedures and physiotherapy.

Oxygen therapy is often a means of averting respiratory failure whilst intensive treatment of the causal condition is undertaken. For example, congestive heart failure responds favourably to rest, digitalis and diuretics; depressed respiration to respiratory stimulants, and haemorrhage to blood transfusion. If, in spite of treatment of the cause, respiratory distress persists or becomes worse, it may become necessary to replace oxygen therapy by mechanical inflation of the lungs, first through an endotracheal tube and subsequently through a tracheostomy.

The theoretical principles and some basic points in the use of mechanical ventilators will be discussed in the next chapter.

Length of Life of an Oxygen Cylinder

The most convenient size of cylinder contains 3,400 litres which lasts a reasonable length of time but is light enough to be handled by one person. The following table gives an indication of at what intervals replacement of a 3,400-litre cylinder will be necessary at various rates of flow.

2 litres per minute	28 hours
3 ,, ,, ,,	19 ,,
4 ,, ,, ,,	14 ,,
5 ,, ,, ,,	11 ,,
6 ,, ,, ,,	9 ,,
7 ,, ,, ,,	8 ,,
8 ,, ,, ,,	7 ,,

HYPERBARIC OXYGEN THERAPY

Theoretical Principles. The exposure of patients to 100% oxygen under pressure in specially designed chambers is known as hyperbaric oxygen therapy. It is a logical development of conventional oxygen therapy since it achieves an increase in the total amount of oxygen carried by the red cells and dissolved in the plasma, thus:

A subject breathing air at atmospheric pressure has only 0·25 ml % of oxygen in solution in the plasma. Breathing *100% oxygen*, besides ensuring complete haemoglobin saturation, raises the amount of dissolved *oxygen* to *2%*. By *doubling the pressure*, the oxygen increases to *4%* whilst at *3 atmospheres* it rises to *6%*, which, in theory at least, is sufficient to meet tissue needs without any red blood cells at all, aptly described by one research worker as 'life without blood'.

Hyperbaric oxygen is a specific form of therapy for carbon monoxide poisoning and infections with anaerobic organisms.

Carbon monoxide poisoning occurs following inhalation of coal gas or exhaust fumes from automobile engines. Carbon monoxide combines with the haemoglobin of the red blood corpuscles to form carboxyhaemoglobin, thus rendering them incapable of carrying oxygen. Oxygen under pressure is of benefit in two ways:

(i) The extra oxygen dissolved in the plasma compensates for the failure of red cells to carry oxygen.

(ii) Oxygen at high pressure displaces carbon monoxide from the red blood corpuscles.

Infection with anaerobic organisms. Anaerobic organisms will only multiply in the absence of molecular oxygen. They occur freely in dead or decaying vegetable or animal matter, and resist drying by formation of spores. They are not uncommonly found in dust, which alighting on moist dead tissues resume active growth. Wounds heavily infected with dirt (e.g. following road accidents) may easily become contaminated. Another source of infection follows criminal abortions performed under unsterile conditions. The organisms produce a lethal toxin and some form gas which spreads through the tissue planes (gas gangrene).

Although hyperbaric oxygen does not *kill* the organism it reduces its activity and production of toxin so that the general condition of the patient improves to an extent which allows the normal defensive mechanisms to deal with the infection.

There are several conditions for which some degree of benefit from Hyperbaric Oxygen is claimed. Treatment has been tried for many disorders of different origin with varying results. Amongst those in which benefit appears to be established are: (i) *Chronic infections resistant* to antibiotic therapy, particularly osteomyelitis (chronic infection of bone) and otitis media (chronic infection of the middle ear). (ii) *Extensive burns*, probably by reducing infection and improving nutrition of the burnt areas. (iii) *Skin grafting* and *organ transplantation* (e.g. kidney grafts). (iv) Certain *forms of cancer*, which may become more susceptible to radiotherapy. (v) *Gangrene* or threatened gangrene from peripheral vascular disease combined with surgical attempts to improve circulation. (vi) The acute stages of *coronary thrombosis*.

Methods of administration. There are two methods of administering hyperbaric oxygen:

1. By means of a *large chamber*, pressurised with air in which the patient breathes oxygen through a mask. This is suitable for certain types of surgery e.g. on the heart or for organ transplant.

2. *Small chambers*, in which the patient is enclosed and which are pressurised with oxygen, are available commercially. Being expensive, they are kept at regional centres to which patients requiring treatment are brought. The chamber consists of a transparent cylindrical shell containing a stretcher which emerges from a hinged door at one end. Operation is semi-automatic from a control panel by a specially trained nurse. The chamber is constantly flushed with oxygen which recirculates after passage through a carbon

dioxide absorber and charcoal filter, thus allowing economic operation.

Complications and hazards of oxygen therapy. There are certain *complications* associated with exposure to high oxygen pressure and *hazards* requiring special precautions. Discomfort and sometimes, pain, may arise from failure of pressure to equalise in the middle ear (a common experience in air travel). The patient should be instructed to swallow or yawn to avoid this complication. Persistent pain may require needle puncture of the ear drum, but is very seldom necessary.

Oxygen increases fire hazards by encouraging combustion and converting a smouldering fire into a blazing inferno, as the Apollo Space Craft disaster illustrated. Special precautions should therefore be taken when using hyperbaric oxygen chambers, to avoid any source of sparks of static origin or from electrical equipment. These have already been discussed on page 90 in the chapter dealing with fire and explosions.

Care of patients. The duration of treatment does not normally exceed 2–3 hours. Even in this short time some patients may become restless from boredom or from claustrophobia. Tranquillisers will help to produce a tolerant attitude.

15 RESPIRATORY FAILURE—III: Ventilators

A ventilator is a machine which inflates the lungs by *positive* pressure through an endotracheal tube or a tracheostomy tube in a rhythmic or 'cyclic' manner resembling normal respiration.

Ventilators were developed as an alternative to tank respirators or 'iron lungs' for long term treatment of patients whose respiratory muscles were paralysed by poliomyelitis. The tank respirator imitated the normal mechanisms of respiration by creating rhythmic *negative* pressure *inside* the tank, in which the patient was enclosed except for the head and neck. The performance of routine nursing procedures presented difficulties, since opening the tank interfered with ventilation.

Positive pressure ventilators, being free from these drawbacks, soon became widely used by physicians for treatment of other forms of respiratory failure, and by anaesthetists to inflate the lungs of anaesthetised patients temporarily paralysed by muscle relaxants. The earlier machines were simple, but with the passage of time those designed for long-term use became more sophisticated by inclusion of controls to *vary the respiratory cycle*; to create *negative pressure* after expiration, and to provide supplementary assistance to patients capable of some respiratory effort by means of a '*trigger mechanism*'. When considering the basic mechanics of ventilators, these additional features can be ignored because all inflate the lungs and produce positive pressure by one of two methods and can be classified as either *volume cycled* or *pressure cycled*.

Volume cycled ventilators are constructed to deliver a *constant volume* to the patient at each inflation. They consist of an electric motor which compresses a bag or bellows containing a *pre-selected volume* of air, at each cycle, irrespective (within limits) of the resistance to inflation.

Pressure cycled (controlled) ventilators are driven by *pre-compressed air* (or oxygen and air) and inflate the lungs until a *pre-selected pressure* is reached when the gas supply cuts out. Pressure builds up again after passive deflation of the lungs through a separate expiratory valve, and so the cycle is repeated.

ADVANTAGES AND DISADVANTAGES OF THE TWO SYSTEMS

Volume cycled (controlled) machines: (i) A *constant volume* is delivered, irrespective of resistance to inflation. (ii) The amount of ventilation is determined by adjustment of the *volume control.* (iii) A *pressure gauge* gives an indication of the degree and changes of resistance to inflation, on the part of the patient or in the circuit. *Decrease of inflation pressure* suggests a leak from a loose connection and that the patient is *not receiving the selected volume.*

Volume controlled machines are preferred for *long-term treatment* because no source of gas is needed, and for patients with chronic lung disease which offers more resistance to inflation. They are larger than pressure controlled machines, are more expensive, and occupy more space at the bedside.

Pressure cycled (controlled) ventilators. (i) Relatively large quantities of *pre-compressed air or oxygen* are required and if piped supplies are not available two or more large cylinders must be kept at the bedside and arrangements made for their replacement when empty. (ii) Adjustment of the *pressure control* determines the amount of ventilation. (iii) A *pressure gauge is not necessary* because the inflation pressure is constant. (iv) A *gas meter or anemometer* on the expiratory side is required to measure the volume of each inflation. (v) If resistance builds up in the circuit ventilation becomes inadequate because the gas supply cuts out when the selected pressure is reached, although full inflation may not have occurred. In the presence of resistance pressure builds up to the limit more quickly and becomes evident from *increase in the rate of cycling.*

Loose connections also *decrease* inflation, but may escape detection because the rate of cycling remains unaltered.

In spite of these disadvantages, pressure cycled machines are widely used and are convenient to use during anaesthesia since a gas supply is readily available.

TREATMENT WITH A VENTILATOR

In most instances the decision to start treatment with a ventilator is taken whilst the patient is still capable of some spontaneous respiration. Unless a tracheostomy has already been performed or an endotracheal tube is in position, a cuffed tube must be passed before treatment can begin, after the pharynx has been made insensitive by a local anaesthetic spray (p. 68).

If the patient is capable of respiratory effort, he may at first 'fight against' the machine, and become exhausted thus defeating the object of the treatment. The following measures are taken to help the patient: (i) Careful adjustment to ensure that *rate*, *volume* and *phasing* are correct to ensure comfort. A doctor familiar with the machine is best able to accomplish this.* (ii) Calm encouragement and assurance to secure confidence and co-operation, a task for which a nurse is particularly well qualified. (iii) The use of drugs which calm the mind and reduce respiratory effort.

Tranquillisers (p. 190) are used to encourage toleration—phenothiazines (promazine—'Sparine', or chlorpromazine—'Largactil') or diazepam—('Valium').

Opiates reduce respiratory effort by depressing the respiratory centre (p. 121), a predominant effect of phenoperidine ('Operidine') and fentanyl ('Sublimaze'). Once the patient is able to tolerate the machine, hyperventilation induces sleepiness and reduces respiratory effort so that prolonged administration of opiates becomes unnecessary and the hazard of addiction is avoided.

Patients on ventilators should be treated in an Intensive Care Unit and their nursing care is discussed in Chapter 19.

Negative phase. Some ventilators have a device to produce 'negative' or subatmospheric pressure during the expiratory phase, in order to increase venous return to the heart. The figure of 5 cm water should never be exceeded for fear of producing oedema of the alveoli. When chronic lung disease is present, negative pressure can be harmful and should not be used unless specific instructions are given.

* The *rate* should be 15–17 per minute, but higher rates are required for patients with pneumonia and for children.

The volume of each inflation should be between 500 and 700 ml. The volume per minute is the rate multiplied by the volume of each inflation and should be between 6 and 11 litres per minute. It is better to err on the side of excess, but if there is any doubt due regard should be given to the subjective feelings of the patient whose personal comfort is the best guide. All patients should in any case be hyperventilated because of the increase in physiological 'dead space' (p. 121) and because the lowered carbon dioxide content of the blood contributes to tranquillity.

Phasing is the ratio between length of inspiration and expiration. Expiration should be about twice as long as inspiration but shortening inspiration beyond this may result in inadequate expansion of peripheral areas of the lung with patches of collapse (atelectasis).

Trigger mechanism. When normal respiration is to be resumed, a device known as a 'trigger' mechanism will produce inspiration in response to the patient's efforts, thus supplementing them. Co-operation on the part of the patient is essential because all control of rate and minute volume is lost. It is only suitable when the convalescent phase has been reached, and when in use, constant attention is necessary to ensure adequate ventilation.

Humidification. Since an endotracheal tube or tracheostomy are necessary for continued treatment with a ventilator, the normal mechanism whereby inspired air is warmed and moistened by passage through the nose and pharynx is lost. Drying and crusting of secretions may occur which defy suction unless some method of supplying warm moist air is included in the circuit. The simplest and most effective humidifier is a water bath, kept at a temperature of 40–60° C, through which the inspired gas passes before reaching the patient at a temperature of 27–32° C and 80% saturation.

A nebuliser, which produces a fine 'mist' of moisture, is an alternative way of providing humidification, and some ventilators are fitted with one for use when desired.

CLASSIFICATION OF SOME VENTILATORS IN GENERAL USE

Pressure cycled	*Volume cycled*
The Bird	The Beaver
The Barnet	The Blease 500 and 4050
The Cyclator	The East Radcliffe
The Manley	The Smith Clarke
The Minivent (pocket size)	The Cape Waine
The Takaoka (pocket size)	

The Barnet ventilator and Blease pulmoflator can be adjusted to operate either as pressure or volume cycled machines.

16 RESPIRATORY FAILURE—IV

A tracheostomy is a rounded aperture cut in the upper end of the trachea just *below* the cricoid and thyroid cartilages (the Adam's Apple) which enclose the vocal cords (Fig. 54).

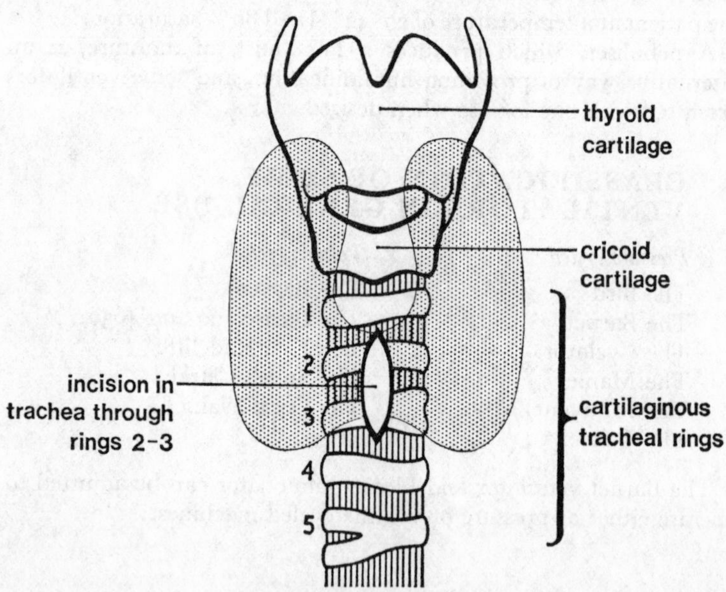

Fig. 54 Site of tracheostomy

INDICATIONS FOR TRACHEOSTOMY

Formerly tracheostomy was almost exclusively an emergency procedure performed to overcome obstruction to the air-way by inflammatory exudate ('membrane') from diphtheria or streptococcal infections. In recent years it has been performed more frequently as a planned proceeding (*a*) in the treatment of *Respiratory Failure*, (*b*) on patients *comatose* from head injuries or cerebral haemorrhage to prevent partial obstruction to respiration from the tongue and aspiration of pharyngeal secretions into the trachea, and (*c*) for patients suffering from loss of nervous control of swallowing (see (v) below).

ADVANTAGES OF TRACHEOSTOMY

(i) Overcomes airway obstruction. (ii) Allows removal of secretions from the trachea and bronchi by suction. (iii) Reduces 'dead space' by about 70 ml (p. 121). (iv) Facilitates mechanically assisted respiration. (v) Prevents aspiration of secretions and food into the trachea in patients with paralysis of the swallowing muscles by separating the larynx from the pharynx.

INSTRUMENTS

The instruments for tracheostomy should always be ready for use in a pre-sterilised pack, which should contain: (i) 2 scalpels, No. 3 and No. 9 handles with size 10 and 15 B.P. blades; (ii) 2 dissecting forceps: fine toothed (Gillies) and non-toothed (McIndoe); (iii) 2 pairs scissors, one curved on the flat and one straight-pointed stitch scissors; (iv) 12 mosquito forceps, 6 straight and 6 curved; (v) 2 7-in straight artery forceps; (vi) 2 single hook retractors—one sharp, one blunt; (vii) 2 double hook retractors; (viii) 2 malleable copper retractors; (ix) self-retaining retractor (mastoid type suitable); (x) tracheal dilating forceps; (xi) metal tracheostomy tubes with introducers; (xii) rubber or plastic tubes with detachable inflatable cuffs (below).

Connections for the ventilator. If a ventilator is to be used an endotracheal adaptor mount and corrugated rubber tube with endotracheal connections will be needed. The Beaver Jointed Connector is a useful form of endotracheal connection when a ventilator is in use because it swivels in a horizontal plane, conferring freedom of movement and minimising the risk of dislodging the tube.

Tracheostomy tubes

Tracheostomy tubes are made of *metal* or *plastic* material.

Metal tracheostomy tubes (Fig. 55a) consist of: (i) a blunt-ended introducer; (ii) an outer tube with flanged ends carrying tapes; (iii) an inner tube.

The outer tube is passed through the tracheostomy by means of the 'introducer', which is then removed and replaced by the hollow 'inner tube', which can be removed for replacement or cleaning without disturbing the outer tube which remains in position for 5–7 days to allow formation of an adequate track.

The inner tube is changed frequently (half hourly) during the early stages because the outer tube itself stimulates secretions which,

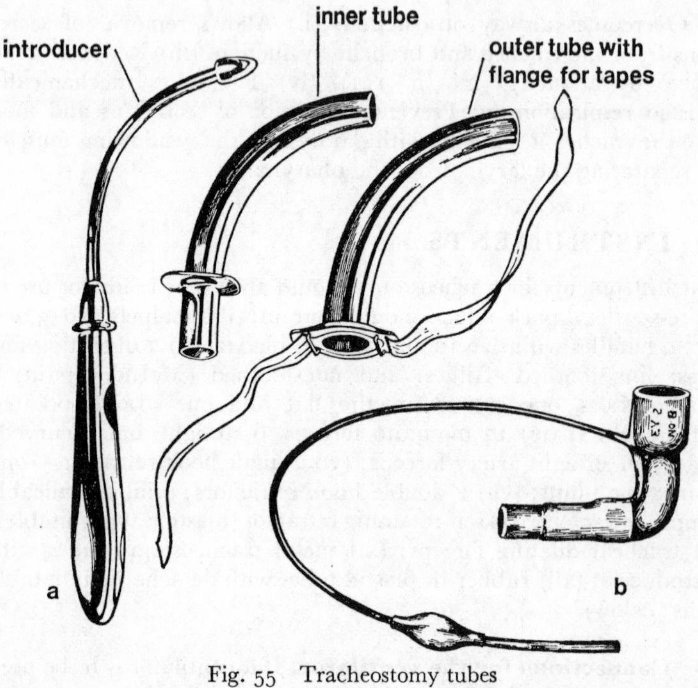

Fig. 55 Tracheostomy tubes
a metal b cuffed latex

together with blood from the wound, dry forming crusts on the inner tube, preventing free flow of air.

Plastic tubes. If mechanical ventilation is necessary, or there is need to prevent inhalation of pharyngeal secretions from disorders of swallowing, a nylon reinforced tube with an inflatable cuff is used.* These are of two types: (i) *The right-angled tube* (Fig. 55b). The right angle reduces the risk of the tube slipping out. (ii) *The Portex disposable latex tube*, which is curved and the one usually preferred.

* Rubber tubes are no longer used because they irritate the trachea.

Securing the tracheostomy tube. After insertion, the tube is secured by passing the tapes attached to the flange round the neck and tying them in a single bow knot with short loops and long ends. They should be tied as firmly as is compatible with comfort, but without obstructing the venous return in the neck.

OPERATIVE TECHNIQUE

Tracheostomy is no longer classed as an emergency unless respiratory obstruction cannot be relieved by passage of an endotracheal tube.

Position of the patient. The operation is more difficult if the patient's head is not in the correct position. The head should be slightly extended by placing a *small* flat sandbag under the back of the neck, and in line with the neck in the horizontal plane. Deviation to one side distorts the normal anatomy so that it may be difficult to locate the trachea. A small sandbag on either side of the head lessens the possibility of inadvertent movement.

Children. As it is sometimes difficult to locate the trachea in children, a small bronchoscope may be passed, since its light is a useful guide. This instrument should be prepared for use when the operation is on a child.

Anaesthesia. General or local anaesthesia may be used. When general anaesthesia is chosen, the anaesthetic hose is transferred to the tracheostomy tube as soon as it is in position. The correct fitting *mount* and connections should be assembled beforehand with *towel clips* and *tape* to secure the anaesthetic hose and avoid dislodging the tube.

If the operation is not carried out in the intensive care unit, the patient should be moved there as soon as possible. Artificial ventilation is needed during the transfer by means of an Ambu bag or Cardiff bellows (p. 150). The subsequent care of the patient with a tracheostomy will be considered in the next chapter.

17 RESPIRATORY FAILURE—V:

MAKING CONTACT WITH THE PATIENT

Patients with a tracheostomy are unable to talk and can only communicate by signs or by writing. A pen and paper should always be within easy reach of the patient and a watch kept for small movements of face or hands which might indicate a request. An explanation of what is to be done and why it is necessary should always precede touching or disturbing the patient. This will make certain that the patient is awake; ensure co-operation, and relieve any anxiety to which a sudden move or change may give rise.

GENERAL CARE

There are several important details which should receive attention.

(i) All connections must be kept firm and tight to prevent any leakage of air.

(ii) The corrugated rubber breathing tubes will require emptying half hourly because considerable condensation of water occurs since the gases are saturated with water vapour.

(iii) The connections between the ventilator and the patient should be well supported with towel clips or slings so that the breathing tubes do not drag on the tracheostomy tube.

(iv) The tracheostomy wound dressing will require changing every *four hours*, preferable after physiotherapy (p. 144). Gauze soaked in 1/2000 Hibitane will keep the wound free from infection.

(v) *Deflation of tracheostomy cuff.* In some units the cuff of the tracheostomy tube is deflated for five minutes every four hours, in others once the cuff has been inflated it is left undisturbed and only changed once a week. *Deflation* of the cuff is carried out as follows: (*a*) the head is lowered before deflation to prevent secretions running into the trachea when the cuff is deflated. Any secretions are sucked out from the back of the throat. (*b*) The cuff is deflated for five minutes, reinflation being preceded by suction. Only the minimum pressure of reinflation to prevent air leaking back around the tube should be used. (*c*) After reinflation tracheal suction should be performed. Should there be any difficulty, the tube should be changed.

Periodic deflation is advocated by those who maintain that uninterrupted pressure of the cuff on the tracheal mucosa damages the epithelium, and causes infection and narrowing (stenosis) of the trachea. *Those who oppose periodic deflation* assert that no damage is caused if the cuff is properly placed and only inflated sufficiently to prevent leakage of air. They consider that periodic deflation disturbs the patient and induces a bout of coughing, which moves the tube and damages the tracheal mucosa and that malposition of the tube may occur during reinflation.

ENDOTRACHEAL SUCTION

A bed-ridden patient with a tracheostomy, even if conscious, cannot expectorate. Secretions, unless removed from the trachea by suction, will accumulate and interfere with ventilation which become evident from a rising pulse rate and blueness (cyanosis) of lips and finger tips. The frequency with which suction should be performed depends on the quantity of the secretions. When copious, suction may be necessary every quarter of an hour; when less, the interval can be longer, for example, up to one hour. It is impossible to lay down hard and fast rules. When in doubt the best advice is to perform suction since it is better to err on the too frequent side.

Equipment for tracheal suction. Before starting suction the following equipment is required:

(i) *A source of suction set* at low vacuum, together with pressure tubing and a plastic or metal sucker end (p. 52) which should be immersed in 1/2000 aqueous Hibitane solution until needed.

(ii) *Sterile suction catheters.* There are several types, the Franklin whistle-tipped catheter is widely used.

(iii) *Sterile 5% sodium bicarbonate solution* to lubricate the catheter and loosen dried secretions in the trachea.

(iv) *Two sterile dissecting forceps* to hold the catheter unless sterile gloves are worn.

Performance of tracheal suction. Scrupulous aseptic technique must be followed to avoid introduction of infection into the trachea and air passages. An assistant is needed to disconnect the ventilator before suction and re-connect afterwards. Suction must be carried out expeditiously in order to minimise interruption of oxygen supplies, and the ventilator *should never be disconnected from the patient for more than twenty seconds.* (i) After 'scrubbing up', a catheter is removed from its covering with sterile forceps, and dipped in the sodium bicarbonate solution. (ii) The suction tubing is nipped to close off the suction and the catheter connected to the suction end. (iii) An assistant disconnects the ventilator, and with the tubing still nipped the catheter is inserted by means of the forceps* to its fullest extent into the trachea. (iv) The tubing is released and suction maintained whilst the catheter is withdrawn from the trachea. (v) The assistant reconnects the ventilator as soon as the catheter is withdrawn.

If secretions are copious the procedure can be repeated three or four times, allowing an interval of 30 seconds between each operation, and using a fresh catheter on each occasion.

Note. The suction tubing is nipped *before* insertion to prevent the suction of airborne organisms into the catheter and *during* insertion to avoid sucking oxygen from the air passages.

The amount, colour and type of sputum obtained should be noted in the patient's record. The *colour* may be '*white*', '*yellow*', or '*blood stained*'; the *type* may be described as '*frothy*', '*mucoid*', or '*watery*'.

CHEST PHYSIOTHERAPY

The object of chest physiotherapy is to encourage the movement of secretions from the deeper parts of the lung to the bronchi so that a suction catheter can remove them. There are two methods: (*a*) 'Rib springing' or 'vibration' and (*b*) 'percussion' or 'clapping' of the chest wall. Both procedures mobilise secretions in the deeper parts of the lungs and their onward progress is aided by the activity of the cilia (fine hairs) of the epithelial cells which line the air passages.

(*a*) *Rib springing or vibration* consists of placing the palms of both hands flat over the lower ribs and making a few sharp shaking movements.

(*b*) *Clapping or percussion* of the chest is performed by placing one hand palm down over the ribs and striking the back of it sharply two or three times, with the other hand.

During intervals between physiotherapy periodic observation of chest expansion will reveal whether it is full and equal on both sides. Unequal movement of the chest is an indication of need for suction. *Obstruction from accumulated secretions is a common cause of oxygen lack and difficulty in breathing.*

* If sterile gloves are worn it is not necessary to hold the catheter with forceps.

GENERAL NURSING CARE

The general principles of nursing care of seriously ill patients in Intensive Care Units are discussed on page 159. These apply with equal emphasis to patients with tracheostomies dependent on ventilators which however complicate the procedures of (*a*) turning and (*b*) feeding.

Turning the patient. The patient should be turned every hour. An assistant is required because *physiotherapy* and *tracheal suction* should be carried out *before and after* turning.

Feeding. Feeding of unconscious, or otherwise incapacitated patients through a Naso-gastric (Ryle's) tube demands special care. (*a*) *Before* feeding the head of the bed should be raised and remain raised for thirty minutes after each feed. (*b*) If food regurgitates from the stomach, feeding should be stopped and pharyngeal suction performed. (*c*) Food should never be given before physiotherapy or changing of the tracheostomy tube. Physiotherapy can induce reflux of food from the stomach. The same danger may occur during the coughing and straining which changing a tracheostomy tube involves with an added hazard of aspiration of stomach contents into the trachea. (*d*) The Naso-gastric (Ryle's) tube should be changed weekly, the fresh tube being passed through the nostril that was previously unoccupied. Injection of an opiate and an anti-emetic will reduce retching and ensure co-operation of an apprehensive subject.

18 CARDIAC ARREST

Cardiac arrest, sudden and unexpected failure of the heart beat, is not necessarily fatal and can respond to treatment when carried out correctly and quickly. It is an emergency which can occur anywhere and at any time of the day or night. First-aid organisations now train their members and the general public in the necessary emergency measures in the hope of maintaining life until the patient can be brought within the scope of the resources of a well-equipped hospital. The chances of saving life following cardiac arrest occurring within the hospital should be much greater but only if (*a*) all grades of nursing and medical staff receive training in the emergency measures necessary, and (*b*) arrangements have been made for a doctor and equipment for supportive treatment to arrive on the scene within 3 minutes of its occurrence. This chapter discusses the causes of cardiac arrest and the organisation of emergency procedures and supportive measures essential for treatment to have a chance of success.

CAUSES OF CARDIAC ARREST

The causes of cardiac arrest are (1) over-activity of the vagus nerve; (2) severe oxygen lack; (3) sensitivity to drugs; (4) degenerative conditions of the blood vessels and nervous tissue of the heart; (5) electric shock.

(1) *Reflex activity of branches of the vagus nerve* which control the heart-beat can cause cardiac arrest when vagal sensory nerve endings are stimulated during simple diagnostic procedures such as examination of the throat, larynx, bronchi, oesophagus or rectum. For the same reason arrest can also occur during radiological procedures from irritant effects of intravenous radio-opaque (impervious to X-rays) solutions injected to detect abnormalities of the kidney (pyelogram); gall bladder (cholecystogram), or blood vessels (angiogram). This mishap has become rare since less irritant solutions have become available.

(2) *Severe oxygen lack* causes cardiac arrest. For example (*a*) asphyxiation by strangulation, drowning, or the aspiration of stomach contents during anaesthesia; (*b*) from respiratory obstruction by laryngeal spasm induced by vomit or blood during recovery from anaesthesia (p. 114), or (*c*) failure of oxygen supplies during anaesthesia due to an 'empty' cylinder or to obstruction of the endotracheal tube by kinking or displacement of the cuff.

(3) *Sensitivity to drugs.* Adrenaline and cocaine stimulate the sympathetic nervous system and may cause cardiac arrest from ventricular fibrillation. Subjects who already have a high adrenaline content of the blood from apprehension are especially susceptible. Patients who have developed a *sensitivity* to drugs ('allergy', p. 184) e.g. penicillin or horse serum, may collapse if they receive a subsequent injection. The condition is known as '*anaphylactic shock*' and is evident from a sudden fall in blood pressure and cardiac arrest. (Intravenous or intra-cardiac injection of adrenaline is an effective antidote).

(4) *Degenerative conditions* of the blood vessels or nervous tissue of the heart: (*a*) *Coronary thrombosis* occurs from the formation of a clot or thrombus which occludes a coronary artery already narrowed by degenerative disease (arteriosclerosis), followed by cardiac arrest from ventricular fibrillation or oxygen lack. (*b*) *Heart block* is the result of degenerative disease of the specialised nervous tissue in the heart (the pacemaker) which initiates and spreads the stimulus for contraction of heart muscle. If the pacemaker fails, cardiac arrest occurs because no stimulus reaches the ventricles. '*Stokes Adams*' syndrome is a condition in which sudden loss of consciousness occurs from this cause, preceded by a convulsive seizure.*

(5) *Electric shock* from high voltage current or lightning can produce cardiac arrest from ventricular fibrillation.

DIAGNOSIS OF CARDIAC ARREST

The events following cardiac arrest arise from oxygen lack which (in the words of the late Professor Haldane) 'not only stops the machine but wrecks the machinery'. The effects of acute deprivation of oxygen supplies are (*a*) immediate loss of consciousness, (*b*) failure of respiration, and (*c*) if untreated for more than three minutes, irreversible damage to the brain cells making full return of consciousness improbable even if the heart does start beating and oxygen supplies are restored.

The diagnosis can be made immediately from the following signs: (i) Loss of consciousness. (ii) Absence of breathing. (iii) Pallor of the

* Artificial 'pacemakers' which maintain the heart beat electrically are often implanted in the chest wall of patients with heart block.

face; blueness of the lips and finger-nails. (iv) Absence of pulsation in the *carotid artery* in the neck.

PRINCIPLES OF TREATMENT

The success of emergency resuscitative measures is wholly dependent on the speed with which they are started after the arrest and this must be within seconds. No special equipment is required and treatment must be undertaken wherever the arrest has occurred. The objects are to maintain respiration and the circulation by *artificial respiration* (using the direct or 'mouth to mouth' method), and by *external cardiac* massage.

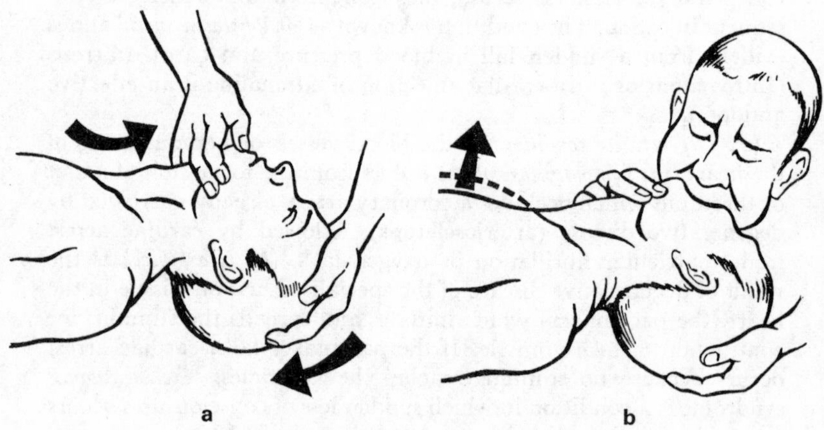

Fig. 56 Mouth to mouth respiration

a correct position of head
b inflation of lungs shown by upward movement of chest

(1) **Direct artificial respiration** by the mouth to mouth method is more effective than the older methods of artificial respiration with which external cardiac massage would be impossible. It is carried out as follows: (i) The patient is placed supine and the throat cleared of vomit or foreign matter, manually or by suction. (ii) One hand is placed under the patient's head tilting it back as far as possible, whilst the other is placed under the jaw pulling it forwards to clear the airway (Fig. 56a). (iii) The operator then pinches the nose and places his open mouth over the patient's mouth (separated if desired by a handkerchief or piece of gauze) and, having taken a deep breath, blows air into the lungs until the chest rises and expands (Fig. 56b). (iv) After a pause to allow expiration (seen by collapse of the chest wall) the process is repeated once every five

seconds until respiration is restored or passage of an endotracheal tube allows manual inflation.

An alternative method of inflation is to breathe through the *nose*, keeping the mouth closed with the hand supporting the jaw. In infants and small children it is possible to blow through both nose and mouth.

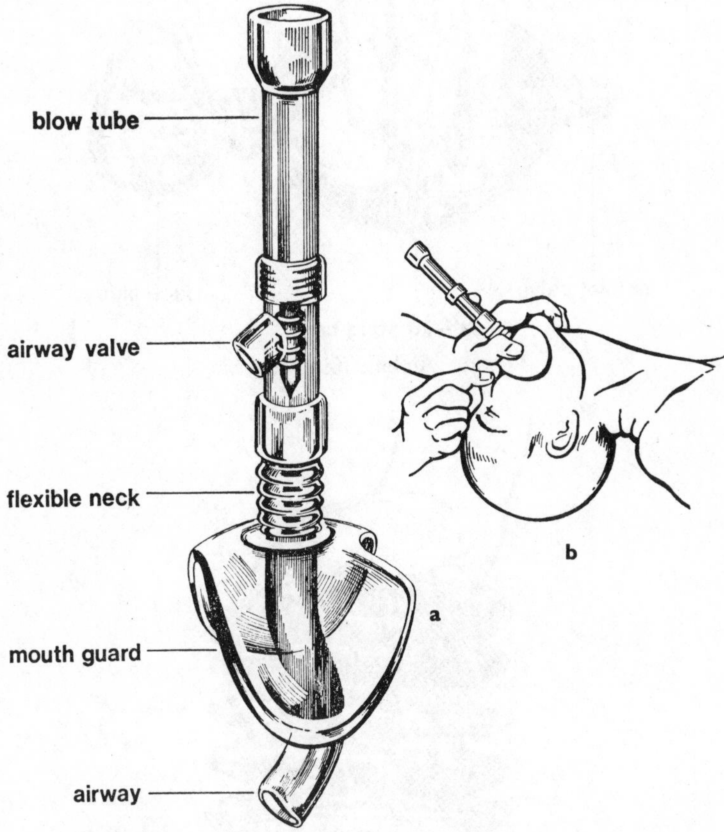

Fig. 57 Brook airway for insufflation of lungs

a Brook airway
b Brook airway in position. The mouthguard is pressed against face and nostrils are pinched to prevent leakage of air.

Direct insufflation should be noiseless—gurgling or snoring are signs of partial obstruction.

Aids to direct insufflation are available, which also overcome aesthetic and hygienic objections to 'mouth to mouth' breathing. They are (*a*) the Brook airway, and (*b*) self-inflating re-breathing bags.

The Brook airway (Fig. 57) consists of a curved airway and mouth-

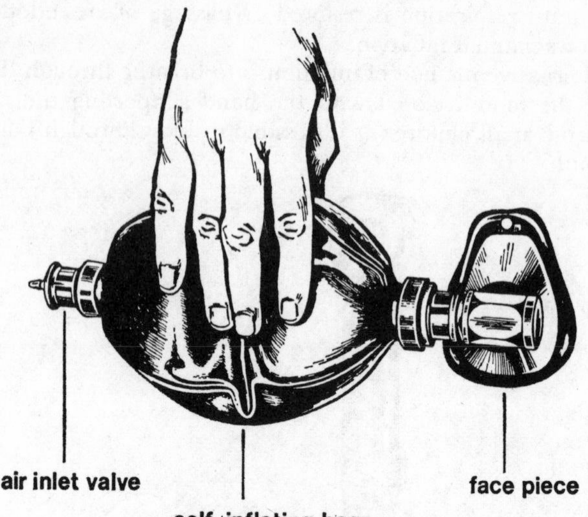

Fig. 58 Ambu self-inflating bag

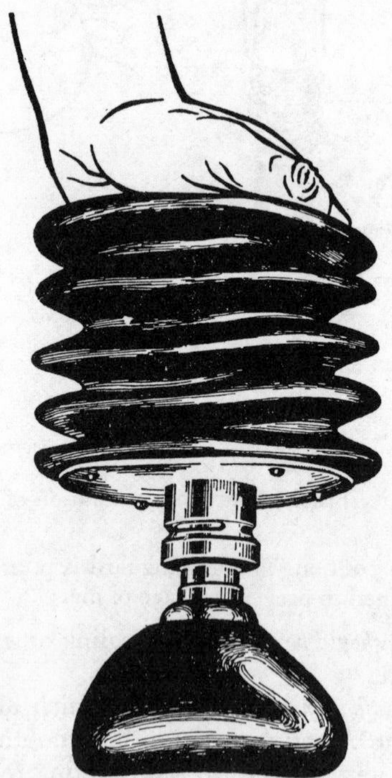

Fig. 59 Cardiff inflating bellows

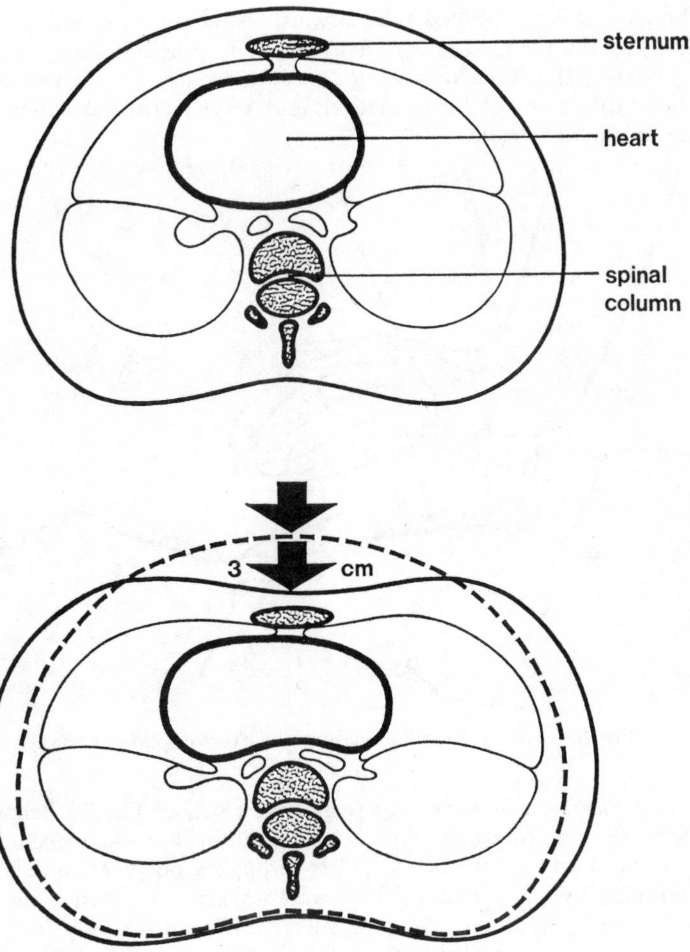

Fig. 60 Mechanism of external cardiac massage. The heart is compressed between sternum and spinal column by depressing the sternum 3-4 cm

guard (to prevent escape of air) connected by a flexible neck to an airway valve and blow tube. The airway is passed over the back of the tongue with the head well extended until the mouthguard rests on the lips. The airway is held in position by grasping it and the chin which is pulled well forward. After pinching the nostrils and pressing the mouthguard against the lips, the lungs are inflated by blowing down the airway once every 5 seconds. The airway valve allows the escape of the exhalations and prevents them reaching the end of the blow tube.

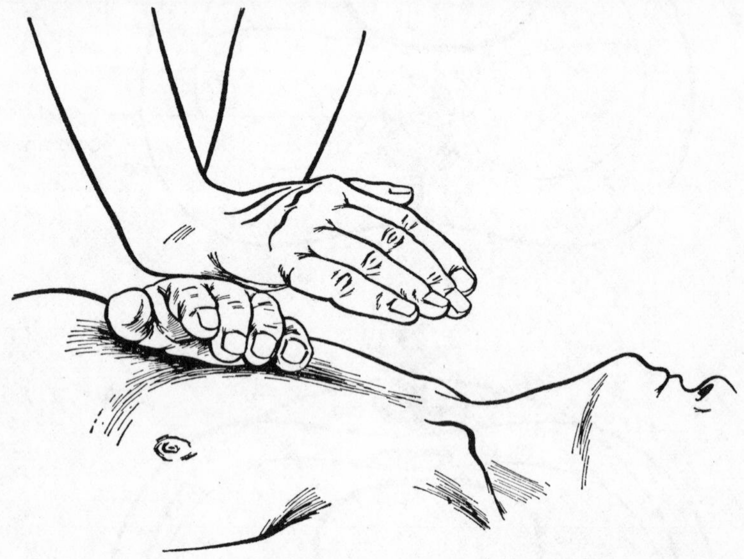

Fig. 61 External cardiac massage—correct position of hands

Self-inflating re-breathing bags (e.g. Ambu bag or Cardiff bellows) (Figs. 58 and 59) are reservoir bags containing a spring mechanism to expand and fill the bag with air through a one-way valve after emptying by compression. They carry a facepiece which is placed firmly over the mouth and nose, after clearing the airway; pulling forward the jaw; and insertion of an oral airway. Rhythmic compression of the bag forces air into the patient's lungs, exhalation taking place through a non-return valve between the bag and the facepiece.

(2) External cardiac massage. The object of external cardiac massage is to maintain the circulation by rhythmic manual pressure on the sternum, compressing the heart between it and the spine and forcing blood into the aorta (Fig. 60). Relaxation of the pressure allows the sternum to rise so that the heart fills with blood. (The older method of opening the chest and compressing the heart by hand, known as 'internal cardiac massage', is no longer practised.) External cardiac massage is carried out in the following way:*

(i) The patient is placed supine on a rigid support. The floor is best for this purpose, but as it is not always possible to transfer a bedridden patient to the floor, a smooth board is provided to slip under the patient instead.

(ii) The operator kneels or stands at the side of the patient, placing the heels of both hands, one on top of the other, over the *lower half of the sternum* (Fig. 61). Aided by the weight of the body, the sternum is rhythmically depressed 3-4 cm and relaxed 60 to 70 times a minute. This should produce a palpable pulse at the wrist and a blood pressure of between 60 and 100 mm Mercury. Excessive pressure on the ribs or the upper part of the stomach should be avoided to prevent fracture of ribs, or damage to the spleen or liver.

ORGANISATION OF TREATMENT FOR ACUTE CARDIAC ARREST

External cardiac massage and direct insufflation are the simple emergency measures designed to maintain life until more sophisticated equipment can arrive whose purpose is (*a*) to maintain respiration more efficiently, (*b*) to restore the heart beat, and (*c*) to counteract the metabolic changes (accumulation of acid waste products, etc.) which occur during the period when the circulation is arrested. Each hospital has its own arrangements, which may differ in detail but basically, emergency treatment of cardiac arrest and/or respiratory failure proceeds in phases.

Phase I—The Emergency Phase. Whoever is nearest to the patient should give the alarm (i.e. instruct an orderly or ambulant patient to alert the hospital telephonist) and collect the emergency apparatus (Brook airway and flat board) which should be kept in a prominent situation in all wards and hospital departments. After clearing the airway, a *strong thump* over the heart may provide sufficient mechanical stimulation to restore the heart beat. If no obvious improvement occurs, cardiac massage and mouth to mouth respiration should be started immediately, an assistant taking over

* It would be reasonable to suppose that the rhythmic compression of the chest during external cardiac massage would move sufficient air in and out of the chest to make direct insufflation unnecessary. It has been shown experimentally that the quantity of air moved in this way is quite insufficient to maintain life. Furthermore, with the patient lying *supine* and unconscious, obstruction of the *airway* by the tongue falling back against the pharyngeal wall (p. 108) is more than likely.

direct insufflation using the Brook airway. *If no assistant is present*, it is advisable to start with *direct insufflation*. If no improvement is seen, then cardiac massage should be done 5 or 6 times, alternating with one insufflation until help arrives.

Phase II—The Supportive Phase. The alarm signal should bring medical assistance. The duty anaesthetist should arrive with equipment (*a*) to perform endotracheal intubation to allow continuation of artificial respiration by manual or mechanical means, and (*b*) to set up an intravenous infusion and administer sodium bicarbonate solution to neutralise acidity, and cardiac stimulants as he thinks necessary. This equipment should be kept ready in a special box (Cardiac Arrest Box) either in the ward or at certain, clearly marked, pre-arranged points near the wards and special departments.

Phase III—The Diagnostic Phase. A Cardiologist will bring (*a*) an Electrocardiograph to diagnose the cause of the arrest and (*b*) A Defibrillator and Pacemaker to reverse electrical disturbance.

Phase IV—Definitive Treatment. Emergency treatment (cardiac massage, direct insufflation, defibrillation, etc.) takes place wherever the arrest occurs. If the heart beat is restored continued observation and special treatment should be continued in the Intensive Care Unit (p. 156) where monitoring facilities, ventilators and constant nursing care are available.

EXAMPLES OF CARDIAC ARREST EQUIPMENT

(1) Emergency Phase. Each ward should have in a prominent position:

(*a*) A Brook Airway.
(*b*) An oxygen cylinder, self-inflating bag and face mask.
(*c*) A flat board to put under patient.
(*d*) Suction apparatus and catheters.
(*e*) Mouth gags (p. 57).

(2) Supportive Phase. Cardiac arrest boxes should be placed at well-marked points convenient for collection 'en route' to the emergency. They should contain:

(*a*) A laryngoscope.
(*b*) Cuffed endotracheal tubes and connections.
(*c*) An endotracheal adaptor mount (p. 66) and rubber tubing.
(*d*) Airways in assorted sizes.

(*e*) An Ambu bag or Cardiff bellows.
(*f*) A 'cut down' set for setting up an intravenous infusion.
(*g*) Intravenous fluids (including 100 ml 8·4% sodium bicarbonate) to reverse 'acidosis'.
(*h*) Cardiac and respiratory stimulants, e.g. Digitalis, Propranolol, Aminophylline, calcium gluconate, vasopressors, etc. and ampoules containing 1 ml of 1/1000 adrenaline.

(3) Diagnostic and treatment. The electrocardiograph, defibrillator and artificial pacemaker may be kept in the Cardiac or Casualty Department or operating suite from whence they can be conveyed to the site of the arrest.

19 THE INTENSIVE CARE UNIT

Advances in medicine and surgery have made it possible to prolong life and cure certain conditions, which formerly were fatal. Coronary thrombosis and respiratory failure can now be treated with a reasonable prospect of recovery and return to home environment. Operations on the heart or blood vessels can restore the function of diseased valves and obstructed arteries. Grafting of kidneys can prolong the life of sufferers from chronic renal disease. These are a few illustrations. But, to ensure success, in addition to skilled nursing, there is need for specialised equipment which is most conveniently kept in a unit set aside for *Intensive Care*.

ADVANTAGES OF AN INTENSIVE CARE UNIT

The advantages of such a unit are: (1) The centralisation of seriously ill patients prevents the dispersal of trained nurses as 'specials' to different parts of the hospital, permits economical deployment of trained staff and increases efficiency of nursing care. (2) Patients in general wards are spared the disturbance and distraction which inevitably arises in the care of seriously ill patients, especially at night, when bright lights are often indispensable. (3) It is possible to concentrate expensive equipment (ventilators, cardiac monitors, suction equipment, defibrillators, etc.) in one place with the certainty that they will be always in a serviceable condition and ready for immediate use.

DISADVANTAGES OF AN INTENSIVE CARE UNIT

(1) Student nurses may not obtain sufficient experience in nursing of acutely ill patients, unless a period of theoretical and practical instruction in the special procedures and nursing principles involved in care of critically ill patients in the I.C.U. forms part of the training

syllabus for every nurse. (2) Since patients leave the ward as soon as the danger period is over, some nurses who work exclusively in Intensive Care experience feelings of frustration because when the critical stage has passed the patient convalesces elsewhere. On the other hand nursing staff in general and convalescent wards miss the satisfaction of successful nursing of critical illness and lack the opportunity to maintain proficiency in nursing skills acquired during their period of training. Some system of rotation would avoid these drawbacks. Any well-trained nurse should be able to undertake intensive care nursing duties. (3) Difficulty may be experienced, in hospitals dealing with large numbers of emergency admissions, in finding a bed in the general wards when the patient is ready for discharge from the unit. The adoption of a system of 'Progressive Patient Care' can help to overcome this by providing greater elasticity in bed occupancy.

GENERAL ARRANGEMENT

Intensive Care Units vary in size according to the number of beds in the hospital, provision being on the scale of 2 beds per 100 patients. The space allowed per patient is about double that allocated in a general ward and each bed has a generous allowance of services, such as piped oxygen, suction, compressed air, and electric points. The general plan is that of an open ward, but cubicles or separate rooms are provided for infected patients, or where quiet and freedom from disturbance are part of the treatment (e.g. coronary thrombosis).

Besides having all the usual offices and equipment of a general ward, the unit has additional features; these are: (1) Laboratory space for carrying out investigations required at frequent intervals e.g. determinating the oxygen and carbon dioxide content, and the acidity (pH) of the blood. (2) Storage space for equipment—ventilators, defibrillators, and cardiac monitors, together with a small workshop for their servicing—either in the ward or close by. (3) Office and sleeping accommodation for the resident doctor. (4) Full air-conditioning.

TYPE OF PATIENT

The criteria for selection of patients varies since the size of the unit often limits the number who can be treated. The following types of illness benefit from treatment in Intensive Care Units: (1) *Multiple injuries*—especially head injuries. (2) Following *major surgery*—especially on the brain, heart, lungs, or large blood vessels. (3) *Treatment for shock*—post-operative, traumatic or haemorrhagic. (4)

Cardiac arrest from any cause, or following a coronary thrombosis. (5) *Respiratory embarrassment*, obstruction to the airway, or respiratory failure from any cause. For example, patients with acute respiratory failure from poliomyelitis and other disorders of the central nervous system; acute exacerbations of diseases of the respiratory system, such as pneumonia superimposed on emphysema, chronic bronchitis and bronchiectasis.

PROBLEMS OF ORGANISATION AND ADMINISTRATION

Administration. Because respiratory problems make up much of the work in Intensive Care Units and ventilators are frequently required, the services of anaesthetists and their assistants are in constant demand so they often undertake responsibility for day to day administration in collaboration with the sister in charge.

Medical supervision. Napoleon is said to have remarked, 'order—counter order—damned disorder!' Often several doctors are concerned with the treatment of the patient. The anaesthetist is responsible for mechanical ventilation; the cardiologist for the heart and circulation; the surgeon for post-operative care; and physicians for other medical aspects. If everyone gives orders, possibly conflicting, the nursing staff can easily become confused, especially if the consultant originally responsible for the patient is not immediately available to give a ruling. In large units it is advisable to delegate to *one person* the duty of conveying instructions to the nursing staff about patient's treatment, which should always be *in writing*.

It is usually agreed that the resident medical officer of the unit is the person to whom various consultants give instructions. He is in the best position to know whether these conflict with each other. Having resolved any differences, if necessary by referral to the consultant with overall responsibility, and thereby achieved unanimity and continuity of treatment, he can convey the decision to the nursing staff.

NURSING CARE IN INTENSIVE CARE UNITS

Taking over the patient. Personal transfer is essential when admitting or discharging patients or when changing duties. The patient's complete record should be available in order that whoever takes over can make a check on all treatments, special procedures and drug therapy together with their respective frequencies. Scrupulous attention to details and the regular performance of special procedures at the *correct time* and an ability of keeping *neat* and *legible* records are the hall-marks of a good intensive care nurse.

General nursing care. The general nursing care of patients does not differ in detail from the nursing procedures necessary for any seriously ill patient in an acute medical or surgical ward, but nurse allocation is more generous, and gives more time for thorough attention to nursing detail. Special attention should be given to turning the patient; treatment of pressure points; cleanliness and dryness of flexures; massage of upper and lower limbs. Passive movements and measures to prevent development of flexure deformities are particularly important when a patient is unconscious. Considerable significance attaches to observation of the adequacy or otherwise of circulatory perfusion (p. 123), which provides a useful indication of the state of the peripheral circulation. The colour of lips or finger nails, bluish or pink; the state of the skin—warm and dry, or moist and cold; the condition of the veins of foot and hand—full or collapsed, are all significant. Accurate observation needs good lighting which does not distort colour.

SOME SPECIAL PROCEDURES

Fluid balance charts. Accurate fluid balance charts (*a*) give information about kidney function, (*b*) allow accurate control of fluid intake. Even a small fluid overload can precipitate cardiac or respiratory failure in patients with no reserve, many of whom have already been resuscitated from failure of these systems.

Total intake and output should be calculated every 24 hours, (e.g. from midnight to midnight or 9 a.m. to 9 a.m. the following day). To be satisfactory a fluid chart should be so arranged that *Intake*, *Output*, *Hourly Balance*, and *Running Total* can be seen at a glance at any hour of the day (pp. 161, 162).

Intake is obtained by adding every hour the sum of the (i) *oral intake*, (ii) *intravenous fluids* and (iii) *blood* (recorded in separate columns) to the *total intake* for the *previous hour*.

Output is similarly calculated by adding each hour the sum of loss (i) in the urine (ii) orally (in vomit and stomach aspiration), and (iii) rectally (in fluid stools)—(also recorded in separate columns), to the previous figure.

The '*Hourly Balance*' is obtained by subtracting *Output* from *Intake*. If *output* exceeds *intake* a '*minus*' sign is placed before the figure, otherwise a 'plus' sign is used. If the hourly balance is negative the figure is subtracted from the last *Running Total* (the sum of all the previous hourly balances) and when positive it is added and entered in the appropriate column.

FLUID BALANCE (excluding blood)

Time	Intake			Output			Hourly balance	Running total
	Oral	Drip	Hourly total	Urine	Oral gastric rectal	Hourly total		Brought forward
12 md	30	0	30	0	0	0	+ 30	+ 30
1 pm	0	30	30	0	0	0	+ 30	+ 60
2 pm	20	120	140	100	0	100	+ 40	+100
3 pm	0	120	120	0	140	140	− 20	+ 80
4 pm	0	100	100	60	40	100	0	+ 80
5 pm	0	0	0	0	100	100	−100	− 20
6 pm	0	100	100	0	0	0	+100	+ 80
7 pm	150	100	250	90	0	90	+160	+240
8 pm	0	50	50	0	20	20	+ 30	+270
9 pm	150	50	200	0	0	0	+200	+470
10 pm	0	250	250	300	0	300	− 50	+420
11 pm								
12 mn								
1 am								
12 md								
			24 h Intake			24 h Output		

Explanation of Fluid Charts

FLUID

i.e. Intake and output of all fluid, orally and intravenously, other than *blood.*

(1) Hourly additions of oral and intravenous fluid are estimated.
(2) Hourly additions of urine, gastric and rectal outputs are estimated.
(3) A plus or minus total is charted.
(4) A 'running total' is brought forward.

Central Venous Pressure. Methods of measuring central venous pressure have already been described on page 85. Central venous pressure estimations are made on patients under treatment for severe shock and after major surgical procedures such as open heart surgery. It indicates the adequacy or otherwise of fluid re-

BLOOD BALANCE

RUNNING TOTAL	Hourly balance	OUTPUT				INTAKE
Brought forward		Hourly total	Peri-cardium	R pleura	L pleura	Hourly totals
+140	+140	60	20	20	20	200
+320	+180	20	20	0	0	200
+320	0	50	10	20	20	50
+350	+ 30	20	10	10	0	50
+250	−100	100	50	0	50	0
+210	− 40	90	40	30	20	50
+310	+100	50	15	15	20	150
+310	0	0	0	0	0	0
+280	−30	30	10	10	10	0
+320	+ 40	60	30	20	10	100
+340	+ 20	30	10	10	10	50
		24 h OUTPUT				24 h INTAKE

BLOOD

i.e. Intake and output of all *blood*.

(1) Hourly additions of all blood transfused—in far right-hand column.
(2) Hourly additions of all blood drained, e.g. via drainage tubes.
(3) A plus or minus total is charted.
(4) A 'running total' is brought forward.

placement after haemorrhage or in treatment of shock from any cause.

It will be recalled that the zero point on the calibrated scale from which venous pressure is calculated should be level with the angle of the sternum or (in some units) the mid-axillary line at the plane of the fourth costo-chondral junction. Adjustment will be necessary whenever the patient is moved or the pillows re-arranged. This can quickly be done by using a long rod with a spirit level attached. One end of the rod is placed on the sternal angle and the other against zero point or the calibrated scale. The zero point is moved upwards or downwards until the rod is horizontal, (as shown by the spirit level) so that zero point and sternal angle are in the same plane.

Normal C.V.P. should be between 6 and 8 ml water. Lower figures indicate need for more fluid, and if more than 10–12 ml too much fluid has been given, or the heart is unable to maintain adequate circulation. Regular observation and recording are therefore essential and any material change should be immediately reported.

SOME CONDITIONS MET IN INTENSIVE CARE UNITS

Cardiac Surgery. Although elective surgery of the heart is restricted to special units, patients with heart wounds may be admitted to any general hospital. The after-care of such patients will be on the same lines as in a special unit. Details can be found in text-books dealing with this subject. The following are some general points:

(i) *Drainage tubes*. Drainage tubes may be placed in both pleural cavities and the pericardium. They will be attached to an under-water seal on suction. They may need frequent 'milking', that is to say squeezing the blood along the tubes in the direction of the drainage bottle.

(ii) *Pressure lines*. Arterial and central venous pressure lines may have been inserted and require constant observation and attention, since material changes in the pressure readings can give an indication of complications. The two commonest are (*a*) reactionary haemorrhage and (*b*) 'Tamponade' i.e. filling of the pericardium with blood, and causing cardiac embarrassment. In either event rapid deterioration of the circulation will occur with a rise in pulse rate, fall in blood pressure and a rise in central venous pressure.

(iii) *Ventilators*. The patient may be maintained on a ventilator for 24–48 hours after operation. This ensures adequate ventilation and spares expenditure of energy necessary to do the work of breathing.

(iv) *Monitoring*. Regular blood gas analysis, and constant recording of the electrocardiogram will be undertaken. Instructions in reading an electrocardiogram is given in most units. Multi-channel electronic monitors are now in use which provide a simultaneous visible record of electrocardiograph, blood pressure and venous pressure. Besides making observation simpler less accumulation of equipment is necessary round the patient's bed as all the leads to the monitor can be placed in one cable.

Coronary Thrombosis. Complete rest is the keynote to treatment, which is often carried out in a cubicle or side room. It is usual to nurse in the sitting position because lying flat may induce breathlessness.

Monitoring. Excessive zeal in monitoring may not always be beneficial for the patient. A constant audible 'bleep' with each heart beat can become a source of anxiety to someone who has had a severe heart attack or cardiac arrest. Sudden automatic inflation of a blood pressure cuff can disturb and even frighten a patient who has just dozed off to sleep.

Patients are connected to an electrocardiograph with recording facilities in the same way as patients after open heart surgery, but constant recording should not always be necessary in patients who are conscious, who are past the immediate danger but who are under constant observation. Signs of any adverse change can usually be seen and would be an indication to resume recording.

Blood pressure should *not* be taken too frequently unless there is an obvious change in the patient as indicated by the E.C.G. or deterioration in his general condition because it disturbs the patient. Intravenous fluids are not given as a routine.

Drugs. Coronary patients need treatment for *pain* and *anxiety*. Morphine, Omnopon (papaveretum B.P.), Pethidine and promazine (Sparine) are given for this purpose.

Propranolol ('Inderal') or *intravenous xylocaine* are prescribed to control irregularities of cardiac rhythm, and *digitalis* for heart failure. When digitalis is prescribed, regular charting of pulse rate assumes extra importance since bradycardia (slowing) is a sign of overdose.

Diuretics. Frusemide (Lasix) (p. 186), or *intravenous mannitol* (p. 82) encourage urine flow and overcome fluid retention.

Barbiturate Poisoning. Barbiturate poisoning requires treatment in an intensive care unit when patients are semi-conscious, unconscious, or in respiratory failure. Treatment is as follows:

(i) *Gastric lavage*, preceded, by endotracheal intubation to avoid regurgitation and inhalation of gastric contents during passage of the stomach tube. Fluid aspirated from the stomach must be labelled, sealed and retained for analysis.

(ii) *Blood and urine samples* should be taken and kept for analysis.

(iii) *Intravenous therapy*. An intravenous infusion maintains fluid balance and nutrition during unconsciousness (fluid balance chart will be needed).

(iv) *Hypotension* may require treatment with vasopressors (p. 191).

(v) *Depressed respiration* may require treatment: (*a*) by intravenous injection of respiratory stimulants (p. 190), and (*b*) artificial respiration by means of a mechanical ventilator.

(vi) If there is no response to treatment as indicated by good urine flow, improved respiration and return of consciousness, *peritoneal dialysis* may be undertaken.

Head Injuries. If the patient is unconscious the *first* step is to ensure a clear airway, since some degree of respiratory obstruction is always present and evident as noisy breathing. If the insertion of an airway or adoption of the lateral position do not clear the airway, endotracheal intubation or tracheostomy will be required.

Assessment of the patient. A head injury or 'coma' chart contains the observations required to assess the patient's condition, which should be recorded on admission and at regular intervals and any change being reported immediately. Important points are (i) *level of consciousness*: the patient may be conscious, semi-conscious (i.e. limited response to stimuli) or unconscious (i.e. irresponsive). (ii) *Pulse rate* and *blood pressure* (see below). (iii) *Presence of paralysis*: unilateral or bilateral paralysis of upper and lower limbs may be present and evident from complete flaccidity. (iv) *Pupils*: the state of the pupils, whether dilated or contracted; whether the same or different on each side, are significant for assessment of cerebral damage.

Patients who have been momentarily unconscious before admission and subsequently have recovered their faculties, require careful observation. They may become unconscious once again with a *rise* in *blood pressure* and a *fall* in *pulse rate* (followed later by a rise in rate). These changes arise from increased *intracranial pressure* due to brain haemorrhage for which in certain circumstances, surgery can be a means of saving life. Any such changes in patients under observation for head injuries should be reported to the medical officer in charge immediately.

Hyperpyrexia (high temperature) may follow damage to the heat regulating centres in the brain, and require treatment by artificial cooling with ice bags or an electric cooling blanket. *Chlorpromazine* (Largactil) or *promazine* (Sparine) may be prescribed to prevent shivering and hasten cooling by dilating the skin blood vessels. Temperature is recorded by an electric thermometer placed in the oesophagus or rectum. Regular observation and record is needed because if temperature falls below 32° C cardiac arrest from ventricular fibrillation may occur.

20 LOCAL ANAESTHESIA

Local anaesthesia is a method of rendering surgical operations painless to a conscious patient by the use of drugs known as 'local anaesthetics', which abolish conduction when applied locally to nerve fibres or nerve trunks conveying pain impulses from the operation area. Like general anaesthetics, their action is *reversible* and their use is followed by complete recovery of function without evidence of damage to nerve fibres or cells.

METHODS

There are three methods of producing local anaesthesia: by *surface application*, by *infiltration*, and by *nerve block*.

(1) Surface application. The horny layer of the skin prevents access of local anaesthetics to nerve endings but mucous membranes are only covered by a single layer of cells and can be rendered insensitive by surface application. This method is suitable for examination of the larynx and bronchial tree; to render the urethra insensitive before the passage of bougies or a cystoscope; or to make the conjunctiva and cornea insensitive before ophthalmic procedures.

(2) Infiltration. To produce anaesthesia by infiltration, a dilute solution of local analgesic is injected under the skin surrounding the area of operation. It is a useful method for small procedures such as removal of skin cysts, warts, or a tooth in the upper jaw, and, where there is scarcity of trained anaesthetists, for surgery of the ear, nose and throat.

(3) Nerve block. Nerve block is a self-descriptive term. The transmission of pain impulses is blocked by injecting solutions of local anaesthetics around the nerve trunks supplying the operation area. Examples are:

TABLE 2

	Cocaine	*Procaine* 'Novocaine'	*Lignocaine* 'Xylocaine'	*Bupivacaine* 'Marcain'	*Amethocaine* 'Decicain'	*Cinchocaine* 'Nupercaine'
Surface application	2–10% Nasal paste (20–25%)	No	4%	No	1 mg Lozenges	1 mg Lozenges
Local infiltration	Never	0·5–1% Solution	0·25–0·5%	0·25%	1/2000–1/5000	Not used
Nerve blocks	Never	1–2%	1–1·5%	0·5%	1/500	Not used
Adrenaline for vasoconstriction and slow absorption	Never	1/100,000 to 1/200,000	1/100,000 to 1/200,000	1/100,000 to 1/200,000	1/100,000 to 1/200,000	No
Caudal or Spinal	Never	5% without Adrenaline	Caudal 1·5% with Adrenaline Spinal 5%	Caudal 0·5% with Adrenaline 1/200,000		'Heavy' Nupercaine 0·5% in 6% Glucose 2–3 ml 'Light' Nupercaine 1/1500 in 0·5% Saline, 12–20 ml
Maximum Dose	2 ml 10% 4 ml 5%	0·5–0·8 grammes 500 ml 0·5% 250 ml 1% 125 ml 2%	0·5 grammes 50 ml 0·5% 100 ml 0·25% with Adrenaline	0·15 grammes 30 ml 0·5% 60 ml 0·25% with Adrenaline	0·15 grammes Up to 300 ml 1/2000	3 ml 0·5% 20 ml 1/1500
Duration	Up to 1 hour	30–45 min.	45–60 min.	1–1½ hours	1½–2½ hours	2–3½ hours

(i) *Brachial plexus block.* The arm can be made insensitive by placing local anaesthetic solution around the brachial plexus as it passes under the collar bone. The method is used to allow reduction of fractures of the upper limb, after accidents when general anaesthesia is contraindicated, because the patient has recently taken food or drink with danger of respiratory obstruction from vomiting during induction or recovery.

(ii) *Intercostal block.* The intercostal nerves are readily accessible to local anaesthetic injection as they run in a groove on the underside of the ribs. For extensive operations on the chest wall (e.g. thoracoplasty, removal of several ribs for tuberculosis), the local anaesthetic solution is placed where the nerves emerge from the vertebral bodies and pass under the ribs; a method known as *Paravertebral Block.*

(iii) *Abdominal field block.* The intercostal nerves also supply the abdominal muscles. They can be blocked as they emerge from the ribs along the costal margin and in the space between the ribs and the iliac crest. This technique provides adequate anaesthesia and muscle relaxation for abdominal surgery, when for any reason general anaesthesia is considered undesirable.

(iv) *Nerve blocks for ophthalmic surgery: Supraorbital and intraorbital block.* The branches of the fifth (Trigeminal) cranial nerve can be blocked as they emerge from foramina in the skull above and below the eye, giving anaesthesia of the upper and lower eyelids and the lacrimal gland. *Retrobulbar block:* the nerves to the iris and cornea are made insensitive by injection of local anaesthetic behind the eyeball. *Facial block:* injection around branches of the seventh (facial) cranial nerve at the outer side of the orbit paralyses the upper and lower eyelids and the muscle round the eye (orbicularis oculi). Retrobulbar and facial block, together with surface anaesthesia of the conjunctiva and cornea are used for intra-ocular operations e.g. cataract extraction, iridectomy for glaucoma.

LOCAL ANAESTHETIC DRUGS, THEIR PROPERTIES AND USES

All local anaesthetics, except cocaine, are manufactured synthetically and differ only in the intensity and duration of their actions. Apart from *cocaine,* the local anaesthetics in general use in Great Britain are: *Procaine* ('Novocaine'), *Lignocaine* ('Xylocaine'), *Bupivacaine* ('Marcain'), *Amethocaine, Cinchocaine* ('Nupercaine').

Cocaine is prepared from the coca plant which grows in the South American Andes. The Indians chew the leaves because at high altitudes the sympathetic stimulant effect of cocaine predominates and, like amphetamines at low altitudes, reduces hunger and increases powers of endurance.

Clinical uses. Cocaine is a drug of addiction so is never employed to produce local anaesthesia by injection. Its use is confined to *surface application* to nose and eyes because its vasoconstrictor properties reduce bleeding during surgery. It is also used to induce local anaesthesia of the larynx, trachea and bronchi before endoscopic examinations. Strength of solutions varies from 4% to 10%. Use of high concentrations (strong solutions) is justified on the grounds that the vasoconstrictor action delays absorption of the drug, giving longer and more intense action, whilst lessening risk of toxic effects from absorption into the bloodstream. The *maximum safe dose* is 200 mg, equivalent to *5 ml* of *4%*, *4 ml* of *5%*, and *2 ml* of *10%* solutions.

Toxic effects arise from (*a*) a sympathetic stimulant effect which can cause cardiac arrest, especially in apprehensive subjects, (*b*) The effect of overdose on the central nervous system which causes convulsions and unconsciousness.

Synthetic local anaesthetics. The clinical uses and maximum dosage of synthetic local anaesthetics are set out in Table 1. The *duration* of action varies from just under one hour for *procaine* to three to four hours for *cinchocaine*. Toxicity increases with potency.

Central action of local anaesthetics. The capacity of local anaesthetics to depress nervous activity is not confined to peripheral nerves. Depression of the central nervous system also occurs if concentration in the bloodstream rises. The first effect is drowsiness and insensitivity to pain, an effect which has been exploited by giving intravenous infusions of small amounts of procaine or lignocaine in saline to obtain analgesia after major operations on the chest and abdomen so that deep breathing and chest physiotherapy is less irksome and more effective.

Overdose is evident by restlessness and spontaneous movements of the arms or limbs and unless checked, progresses to convulsions and respiratory failure. Intravenous injection of thiopentone, or diazepam (Valium) is an effective antidote and should always be available when large doses of local anaesthetics are given. Prophylactic premedication with barbiturates reduces the incidence of overdose.

Vasodilator action or local anaesthetics. In contrast to cocaine, local anaesthetics *dilate blood vessels*, so that absorption is rapid and duration of action short. *Adrenaline* added to local anaesthetic solutions, by its vasoconstrictor effect delays absorption and prolongs action. The amount added must be strictly limited, because adrenaline can cause cardiac arrest. One ml of 1/1000 Adrenaline is added to 200 ml of local anaesthetic solution giving a strength of 1/200,000. Adrenaline decomposes rapidly on exposure to the air and should be added *just before use*, the quantity and strength being carefully checked, preferably by the person who makes the injection.

Note. Some proprietary preparations of local anaesthetics, particularly those used in 'cartridge' form for dental anaesthesia, do contain adrenaline, decomposition being prevented by the addition of stabilising substances.

EQUIPMENT FOR LOCAL ANAESTHESIA

The equipment for nerve blocks and infiltration is simple and consists of:

(i) *Syringes and needles.* The Labat syringe (Fig. 62) with needles of varying length, is the most convenient syringe for infiltration, especially when large quantities are to be used. For nerve blocks and procedures requiring small amounts of solution, a sterile 20 ml syringe is adequate, but long needles are necessary when nerve blocks at a depth (brachial plexus block) are to be undertaken.

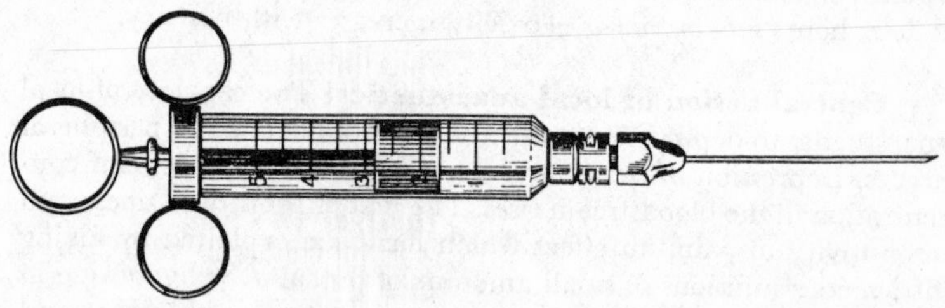

Fig. 62 Labat syringe and needle

(ii) *Antiseptic lotions* for the skin should be *coloured* to distinguish them from the colourless local anaesthetic solution. Plain surgical spirit should *never* appear on the local anaesthetic tray.

(iii) *Sterile towels*, gloves, green gauze swabs (to avoid confusion with the surgical swab count), towel clips and sponge forceps are also required.

(iv) *Local anaesthetic solutions*, a 1 ml ampoule of 1/1000 adrenaline; and a 2 ml syringe and needle (to add adrenaline). The strength of the local anaesthetic solution and the adrenaline ampoule should be checked by the operator (who has the ultimate responsibility for any mistake which may occur in the strength of solutions used) before mixing.

Note. Full aseptic technique should be observed in the preparations and performance of local anaesthetic procedures.

Epidural and Subdural ('Spinal') Anaesthesia

Pre-packed and sterilised equipment for epidural and subdural anaesthesia should include:

(i) Syringes: 2 ml, 5 ml, 10 ml and 20 ml, with hypodermic needles.
(ii) Towels, swabs, towel clips and sponge forceps.
(iii) A galley pot for antiseptic solution.
(iv) Ampoules of local anaesthetic.
(v) A stout needle to puncture the skin (before epidural anaesthesia) or an 'introducer' through which the finer spinal needles can be passed.
(vi) A fine nylon catheter to thread through the epidural needle.
(vii) Specially designed needles for spinal and epidural puncture.

Needles for dural puncture ('Spinal needles') are 7·5–10 cm in length with a narrow bore (20–22 s.w.g.) and carry a fine wire stilette which is withdrawn after successful dural puncture, is evident by the appearance of cerebro-spinal fluid. The Howard Jones needle (Fig. 63a) is an example.

Needles for epidural puncture (Fig. 63) have a larger bore (16–18 s.w.g.) than spinal needles, which makes them appear shorter, though in fact there is little difference in the length. There are several varieties designed to help the accurate placement of the needle into the epidural space; avoid puncture of the dura; and facilitate introduction of an indwelling nylon catheter for repeated injections.

The epidural space contains no fluid. It lies between the tough '*ligamentum flavum*' and the dura of the spinal cord. Loss of resistance and the presence of slight 'negative pressure' transmitted from the thorax, are the only signs that the needle has entered the epidural space. For this reason the *standard epidural needle* (Fig. 63b) has a small mobile bead which can be adjusted to indicate the estimated depth (3–6 cm) of the epidural space.

The Lee extradural needle, a modification of the Howard Jones spinal needle, is calibrated in divisions of 1 cm (Fig. 63c).

The Tuohy needle (Fig. 63d), has a stilette and the orifice on the side to facilitate direction of an indwelling nylon catheter.

Devices are available which, fitted to the caudal needle during puncture indicate that the epidural space has been entered by

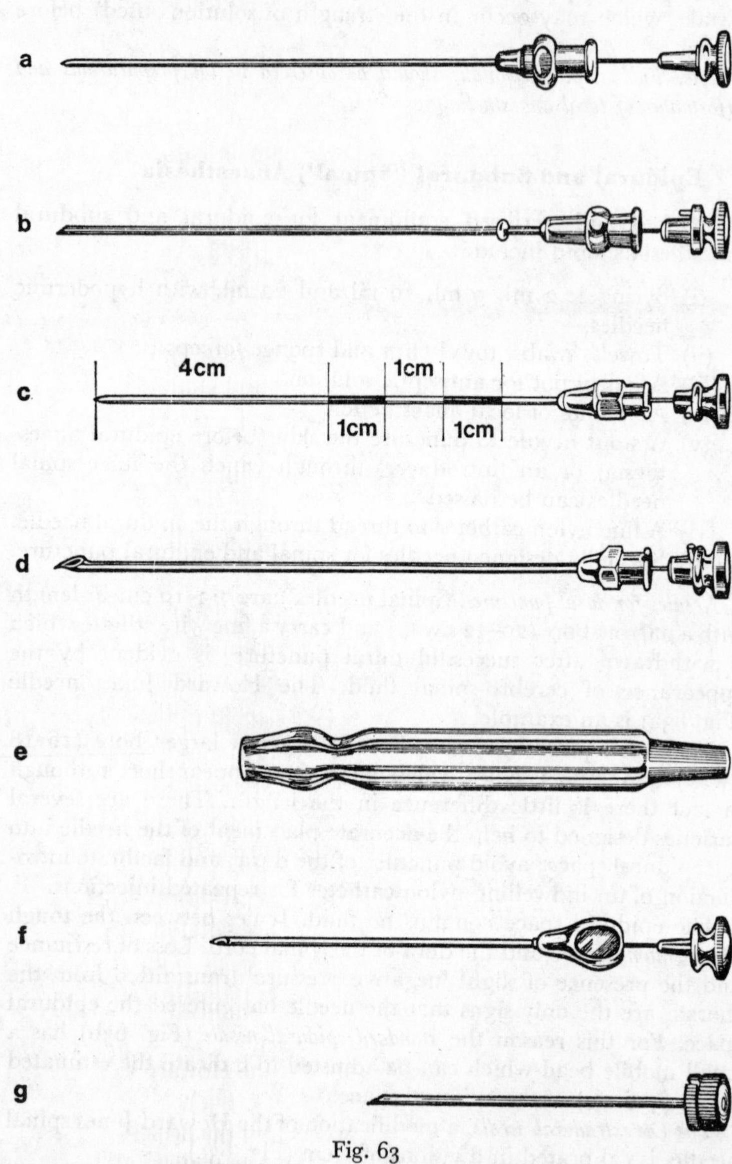

Fig. 63

a Howard Jones spinal needle (7·5 cm 20 s.w.g.)
b Caudal needle with movable bead (19 s.w.g.)
c Lee calibrated extradural needle (20 s.w.g.)
d Tuohy needle (8 cm 16 s.w.g.). Note side opening to aid introduction of nylon catheter
e Odoms epidural indicator
f Magill introducer
g Sise introducer

demonstrating the presence of a slight negative pressure, transmitted from that part of the space in contact with the thoracic cage.

The Odoms epidural indicator is a small glass tube containing sterile coloured water previously injected which on entry to the epidural space (Fig. 63e) is drawn slowly towards the patient.

Another method is to attach to the needle a small latex balloon which collapses on entering the space. Most operators depend on lack of resistance to injection of air from a syringe to indicate successful puncture.

Introducers are short, stout, large bore needles used to penetrate the skin and tough spinous ligaments and through which the finer spinal or caudal needles can be passed. Some (e.g. Magill's introducer, Fig. 63f) carry stilettes. Others (e.g. Sise introducer, Fig. 63g) do not.

Some points in the induction of spinal and epidural anaesthesia. Full aseptic precautions are essential for both procedures, the operators scrubbing up and putting on sterile gowns and gloves. Though important for epidural anaesthesia, the emphasis is even greater when spinal puncture is to be made.

CARE OF PATIENTS

Position of the patient. The *lateral* position is always used for epidural anaesthesia and is convenient for spinal puncture, though for this procedure the *sitting* position is often preferred.

The lateral position. The patient is placed on the side, and an assistant helps to flex the spine in order to open up the intervertebral spaces through which the needle must pass. A co-operative patient can help if asked to try and 'curl himself up into a ball'.

The sitting position. The patient sits up on the operating table with the legs over the side placed on a stool. The assistant should help to keep the spine vertical whilst *flexing* it as much as possible, by keeping one hand on the shoulders and encouraging the patient to flex the head with the other.

On completion of the injection, the patient is turned into the *supine* position, the head made comfortable with pillows, and a screen erected to conceal the operation area. (A slight head-down tilt helps to counteract the effects of any fall in blood pressure (see below)).

Care of the patient during epidural or spinal anaesthesia. Patients under epidural or spinal anaesthesia often receive an intravenous hypnotic injection to induce sleep, e.g. intravenous pethidine and promethazine ('Phenergan') (50 mg of each in divided doses); diazepam ('Valium') or thiopentone. Care must be taken to ensure that the airway does not become obstructed.

Complications. Fall in blood pressure arises from loss of vasomotor tone following paralysis of sympathetic vasoconstrictor nerves by the local anaesthetic. A head-down tilt and an intravenous infusion are common corrective measures. Vasopressors (p. 191) may be needed to restore pressure to acceptable levels. Conscious patients may complain of nausea. The cause is obscure but it has been suggested that increase in vagal tone (often evident by progressive slowing of the pulse) following sympathetic paralysis is a possible cause.

Care of patients during local anaesthesia by nerve blocks or infiltration. Patients are usually ambulant and may not have received any calming or opiate premedication. They should be put in a comfortable position and clothing and coverings arranged to give free breathing and avoid overheating, especially in a warm operating theatre. A comfortable position for the arms is important since their position is often limited by the operation.

Adrenaline added to the local anaesthetics may cause feelings of fullness in the head and a racing pulse. The patient should be re-assured and a pause made to allow the effect to pass off before starting the operation. Faintness and nausea accompanied by pallor, sweating and a poor pulse volume may also arise from over-activity of the vagus, a condition known as the '*vaso-vagal*' syndrome. It responds to lowering of the head to improve blood supply to the brain, and a few sniffs of sal volatile.

The need to *avoid noise* and unnecessary conversation during operations on conscious patients is often forgotten. Careless handling of bowls and instruments jars the patient's nerves and disturbs attempts to relax. Thoughtless conversation of a clinical character can cause unnecessary distress even if it does not concern the individual patient.

21 ANALGESIA AND ANAESTHESIA DURING CHILDBIRTH

Opinions have differed about the need for pain relief during childbirth ever since Dr Grantley Dick Reid in the 1930s asserted that being a natural physiological process it should be painless. He began a campaign, supported by books and pamphlets, to amplify his views that the distress and anguish which many women experienced arose from ignorance of the anatomy and physiology of reproduction and the firmly entrenched belief that pregnancy was abnormal and childbirth dangerous. To overcome what he called 'the fear of the unknown' he urged that all primiparae should receive ante-natal lectures about pregnancy and childbirth together with practical instruction in exercises intended to induce mental and physical relaxation which would render pain relief unnecessary. His methods evoked wide interest and in course of time became known as 'Psychoprophylaxis', or 'Psycho-physical preparation'.

In practice, whilst it has been found that pre-natal instruction is of great value in enabling women to approach childbirth with calm and confidence, it has by no means replaced the need to relieve the pain which many undoubtedly experience during delivery. Current practice in Great Britain divides itself into 2 phases (i) psycho-physical preparation during the ante-natal period and (ii) measures for relief of pain and distress during childbirth.

PSYCHO-PHYSICAL PREPARATION

Psycho-physical preparation is intended for women having their first baby. It consists of a series of lectures during the ante-natal period which cover (i) the *anatomy* of the reproductive organs, the *physiology* of pregnancy and the *mechanisms* of delivery. (ii) Instruction in exercises to encourage *relaxation* of the pelvic muscles and *control of breathing* during childbirth. (iii) Instruction about the analgesia apparatus to be used during delivery.

At some clinics educational talks for husbands are arranged and those who wish to be present with their wives during childbirth may do so.

TREATMENT EARLY IN CHILDBIRTH

Ante-natal instruction helps to induce a calm frame of mind when the moment for admission to hospital arrives. Nevertheless, those experiencing childbirth for the first time may be excited, or distressed and complaining of nausea. At this stage drugs which calm the mind and induce sleep are of more value than those which relieve pain. Drugs with tranquillising and anti-emetic actions like promethazine ('Phenergan') or promazine ('Sparine') will calm the mind and suppress nausea whilst the addition of a barbiturate or chloral preparation will ensure a period of sleep. As labour advances, pain and discomfort increase to a point where relief by an opiate becomes necessary.

All opiates depress respiration and carry a risk of conveying this effect to the newly born child. Various measures are taken to reduce this hazard: (*a*) by the use of pethidine ('Demerol') which depresses respiration less than morphine; (*b*) by simultaneous administration of a phenothiazine (p. 189), promethazine ('Phenergan') or promazine ('Sparine') with pethidine because their tranquillising action increases tolerance of pain and discomfort thus reducing the overall dose of pethidine as well as to some extent antagonising the respiratory depressant effect of opiates; (*c*) by administering intravenously morphine antagonists (p. 187) which reverse the respiratory depressant effect of opiates prior to delivery. Levallorphan ('Lorfan') is used for this purpose. 'Pethilorfan' is a proprietary preparation of pethidine and levallorphan; (*d*) by inducing analgesia by inhalation of anaesthetic vapours during the later stages so that the depressant effects of further injections of opiates within the last hour of delivery is avoided.

ANALGESIA BY INHALATION OF ANAESTHETIC GASES OR VAPOURS

Chloroform was the first anaesthetic used to induce analgesia during childbirth more than 100 years ago by James Young Simpson, a Scottish obstetrician. In spite of opposition on religious grounds by some of his countrymen the method became popular and achieved respectability when Queen Victoria received it for the birth of her third child. Chloroform is no longer administered for this purpose because it can cause sudden death from cardiac arrest and when used for long periods jaundice may occur from liver damage. Less toxic anaesthetics like Nitrous Oxide and Trichlorethylene have been found equally effective. In order to overcome the problems involved in securing the services of an anaesthetist to bring the benefits of analgesia to all patients, apparatus has been designed to induce analgesia by self-administration of nitrous oxide or Trichlorethylene under the supervision of midwives who, however, must receive training in the method and observe certain rules.

APPARATUS FOR SELF-ADMINISTRATION OF NITROUS OXIDE

There are two types of apparatus for self-administration of nitrous oxide, the 'Minnitt' and the 'Entonox'.

Minnitt's apparatus delivers a mixture containing 50% nitrous oxide and 50% air, intermittently on 'demand' from the patient. The apparatus was designed by Dr R. J. Minnitt, Liverpool Royal Infirmary.

It consists of (i) two cylinders of nitrous oxide (one 'full' and one 'in use') connected to a reducing valve which delivers nitrous oxide at 15 lb per sq. in to (ii) a reservoir bag with a lever on the outside which compresses the neck of the bag as it fills with gas and shuts off the gas flow when it is full.

When the patient inhales, a check valve near the mouth of the bag opens and gas flows, entraining air through perforations on the side of the metal mount carrying the breathing hose, to provide a mixture of 50% nitrous oxide and 50% air. Although oxygen content is reduced 20% to 10%, and constitutes a theoretical objection to the method no harm ensues mother or child because inhalation is intermittent.

The 'Entonox'. The reduction of available oxygen when inhaling nitrous oxide and air has been overcome by administering a mixture of 50% nitrous oxide and 50% oxygen pre-mixed in one cylinder from an apparatus known as the 'Entonox'. Although nitrous oxide under pressure is *liquid* (p. 32) it *dissolves* in oxygen and the mixture becomes gaseous so that the pressure gauge gives an accurate indication of the contents (see also p. 34). The 'Entonox' is a simple device consisting of a single unit comprising a *reducing valve*, *'sensing' diaphragm* and *flow control* valve with breathing tubing and facepiece which is attached to a cylinder of *pre-mixed gases* with a pressure gauge. When the patient inhales, the 'sensing' diaphragm opens the flow control valve which delivers the mixed gases at a rate sufficient to meet the demands of a person breathing at *six times* the normal rate thus making a *reservoir bag unnecessary*.

APPARATUS FOR SELF-ADMINISTRATION OF TRICHLORETHYLENE

Although 0·5% trichlorethylene vapour in air is sufficient to induce analgesia, and can be obtained by drawing air through a small glass inhaler containing the liquid anaesthetic, such inhalers are not satisfactory for use without medical supervision because the concentration delivered increases when the temperature in the surrounding air rises.

Temperature controlled inhalers from which a constant percentage of vapour within a wide range of temperature can be assured are however approved by the Central Midwives Board for use by midwives without medical supervision. They are known as the '*Tecota*' and '*Emotril*' temperature compensated inhalers. The quantity of air which is drawn over the liquid on inhalation is regulated by a metal rod carrying a flat valve. When temperature rises, the rod expands tending to close the valve and reduce the amount of air passing over the liquid. When temperature falls, the rod contracts admitting more air so that whatever the temperature the concentration delivered to the patient is always 0·5%. Each machine is checked annually to ensure accuracy by the National Physical Laboratory who issue a certificate which must be kept with the inhaler.

ANALGESIA BY INHALATION DURING DELIVERY

Unless instruction has been given in the ante-natal clinic, the patient should be shown the apparatus and told how to use it as soon as possible after admission. The following points should be emphasised: (*a*) that an *interval of 15 seconds* will occur *between the first inhalation and onset of analgesia*, to allow time for the anaesthetic to enter the circulation and reach the pain areas in the brain, and (*b*) that pain relief occurs without loss of consciousness.

Checking the apparatus. Although after each use the apparatus should be left ready for use by the next patient this practice is often neglected in the excitement following delivery and a second check before use is essential. An 'empty' cylinder should be replaced on the Minnitt's apparatus, and a 'full' spare cylinder be ready for the 'Entonox'. Trichlorethylene inhalers should be 'topped' up.

Choosing the face mask. For the success of the method the face mask must fit the face snugly and be held firmly in place, otherwise air will be drawn under the sides of the mask diluting the vapour, with consequent failure to obtain good analgesia.

Method of administration. The method of administration depends on the stage of delivery.

(i) *Before full dilation of the cervix, inhalation should take place during uterine contractions.* In order to gain maximum benefit it should *start about 15 seconds before each contraction*, since it takes this time for the vapour to reach the brain. With experience it is not difficult to anticipate the onset of a pain, and beginners can observe intervals with a watch or by the second hands of the clock. During intervals between contractions the patient should relax and remove the mask from the face.

(ii) *When the cervix is fully dilated*, the patient has to bear down or push the baby onwards during contractions, and to do so must hold her breath. Inhalation should take place in the interval between contractions and stop at the onset of a contraction. Analgesia remains effective because the anaesthetic remains in the circulation whilst breathing is suspended.

(iii) *During the actual birth of the child* inhalation is continuous to provide maximum analgesic effect.

MAIN FACTORS FOR SATISFACTORY ANALGESIA

1. *Educational lectures* during the ante-natal period, including practical instruction in the use of analgesia apparatus.
2. Ensure the *apparatus is in working order* before use.
3. *Selection of a mask that fits properly* making sure the patient knows how to hold it firmly on the face.
4. *Before full dilatation*, begin inhalations *15 seconds before the onset of contractions* and continue until the uterus relaxes.
5. *After full dilatation* inhalation *between contractions* in order to be able to hold the breath and push down during contraction.

LEGAL REQUIREMENTS

The following regulations have been laid down by the Central Midwives Board and must be fulfilled before a midwife may administer analgesia from a recognised apparatus without medical supervision.

1. Attendance at a course of lectures by a consultant anaesthetist on the theory and practice of administration of anaesthetics to induce analgesia during labour.

2. Practical instruction in the use of the analgesia apparatus under supervision.
3. Before administering analgesia a written certificate that the patient is physically fit must be obtained from the doctor in charge.
4. A third party must be present during the whole period of the administration, to assist if restlessness occurs during analgesia and to protect midwives against allegations of misconduct during the delivery.

ANAESTHESIA DURING CHILDBIRTH

General, *Local* or *Regional*—Anaesthesia is administered for the following procedures.

1. Induction of childbirth by artificial rupture of the membranes.
2. Forceps delivery.
3. Caesarean section; before childbirth begins ('elective' section) or for complications arising during delivery e.g. distress, accidental haemorrhage, placenta praevia, toxaemia.
4. Manual removal of the placenta.
5. For 'stitching' the perineum.

General anaesthesia. The apparatus and equipment required for general anaesthesia has already been described.

As, however, anaesthesia is often needed quickly (e.g. foetal distress or maternal haemorrhage) a tray or trolley with drugs and equipment should be kept ready for immediate use at any time. A 'cut out' on the top of the anaesthetic table or syringe trolley with inserts labelled for each item allow a quick check before use and simplifies re-stocking afterwards. No anaesthetic should be attempted in the labour ward without suction apparatus ready for immediate use.

HAZARDS OF GENERAL ANAESTHESIA FOR OBSTETRICS

The risk of vomiting or regurgitation of stomach contents is greater during obstetric anaesthesia than during routine procedures because patients become thirsty and may drink freely during long delivery and those admitted for emergency procedures may have eaten a recent meal. Furthermore, analgesic drugs and the excitement of childbirth delay the emptying of the stomach. The following measures are recommended to reduce risks of anaesthesia with a full stomach:

(i) Patients should drink sparingly, and then only water, during the later stages. (ii) One ounce of magnesium trisilicate mixture (a strong alkali which neutralises acid gastric juice, the cause of fatal lung damage from inhaled vomit) should be administered hourly. (iii) Enquiry should be made about the time of the last meal from all patients admitted for an emergency obstetric operation.

LOCAL ANAESTHESIA

Local anaesthesia avoids the hazards of general anaesthesia to the patient and the possible depressant effects on the child of the drugs used. Two main methods are available.

1. *Pudendal block.* Local anaesthesia by block of the pudendal nerves as they enter the upper part of the vagina is an alternative to general anaesthesia for forceps delivery and perineal suture. The preparations have already been described in Chapter 20.

2. *Continuous epidural block.* Abolishes all sensation in the lower part of the body during child birth. Analgesia is induced through a nylon catheter placed in the epidural space. Additional topping up doses of local anaesthetic can be given through the catheter as required as child birth proceeds.

Advantages claimed for this technique are: (i) Since opiate analgesics which depress respiration are not required, no problems arise in the breathing of the new born child. (ii) The patient is able to co-operate during delivery. (iii) Birth is painless.

Disadvantages are: (i) Paralysis of the pelvic muscles disturbs the normal mechanism of labour. The foetal head does not rotate and remains in the posterior position requiring application of forceps for delivery. (ii) The progress of childbirth often becomes slower. (iii) A fall in blood pressure from blockage of sympathetic nerves may require administration of vasopressors (p. 191). (iv) Infection of the puncture site is an occasional complication.

Experience in large obstetric units has demonstrated that in capable hands the advantages of epidural analgesia far outweigh the disadvantages, most of which can be anticipated and overcome provided that those who carry out the procedures have adequate training and experience. This method has increased rapidly in popularity during recent years and all large obstetric units now provide an epidural service for those patients who require it.

22 DRUGS AND THEIR USES

Thirty years ago the number of drugs used in Anaesthesia could be counted on the fingers of one hand. Today they are numerous enough to justify a separate textbook, and the task of recognition is complicated by the existence of two or more often dissimilar names for each preparation (Proprietary names and Approved names). No-one expects nurses or theatre technicians to be masters of clinical pharmacology, but it is a considerable advantage to have a knowledge of the purpose for which drugs are intended and the occasions on which they are used.

The Therapeutic Index set out in the form below is an attempt to provide a quick and easy way of supplying such information. It is not intended that it should be read from start to finish at one sitting but used rather as a source of reference when unfamiliar preparations are encountered.

Whenever possible the *Proprietary* and the *Approved* name are given. Where the preparation is discussed more fully in the text, the number of the relative page is indicated for further reference.

Note. The *Proprietary name* of a drug is that given by the Pharmaceutical manufacturer. The first letter is printed with a capital letter. An *Approved name* is (that) approved by the British Pharmacopœia and is printed without a capital letter. The name indicates the chemical composition, but when this is complicated and lengthy an abbreviated form is used.

Adalin'—Carbromal—non-barbiturate hypnotic (see Hypnotics).

Adrenaline ('Epinephrine U.S.P.')—Active principle of the medullary part of the adrenal gland. Liberated with nor-adrenaline at sympathetic nerve endings. Amount circulating increased by fear and apprehension—sometimes called 'Emergency' hormone. Increases heart rate, raises blood pressure, constricts skin vessels, dilates blood vessels in muscles and bronchiolar muscles.

Uses

(i) Added to local anaesthetic solutions (1 ml of 1/1000 to 200 ml = 1/200,000) to delay absorption by vasoconstrictor effect (p. 170) and in similar proportion to normal saline for subcutaneous injection to reduce bleeding during operations under general anaesthesia—(Thyroidectomy, perineal repair).

(ii) Injected directly into heart after cardiac arrest (p. 155).

(iii) Antidote for anaphylactic shock (p. 147) and relief of allergic states, especially asthma (Bronchospasm).

Adrenergic Drugs—Have an adrenaline-like action and are used to raise blood pressure (*see Vasopressors*).

Adrenolytic Drugs—Antagonise the action of adrenaline and nor-adrenaline at sympathetic nerve endings. Commonly prescribed for treatment of high blood pressure. Fall in pressure may occur if patients receiving them undergo anaesthesia (p. 18).

Alloferin (see Toxiferene).

Amethocaine—Long acting local anaesthetic (p. 167).

Aminophylline—Relaxes smooth muscle of bronchi—effective against asthma and bronchospasm during anaesthesia.

Amphetamines ('Benzedrine')—Adrenergic drugs with central nervous stimulant action (see Vasopressors).

Amyl Nitrite—Aromatic and volatile liquid smelling of pear-drops, prepared in capsules. Inhalation from a crushed capsule relieves muscle spasm, e.g. 'Anginal' pain, uterine cramps, hiccough.

Amylobarbitone ('Amytal')—Barbiturate hypnotic (see Hypnotics).

'Amytal'—See Amylobarbitone.

Analeptic—Respiratory stimulant for treatment of depressed respiration,

(*a*) during anaesthesia and recovery.

(*b*) during respiratory failure from *any cause*.

Analgesics—Drugs for relief of pain. Two types—(i) *addictive*, (ii) *non-addictive*.

(i) *Addictive analgesics*—Derivatives of opium and synthetically prepared drugs with similar chemical composition. All carry danger of addiction, and therefore only used to treat *severe* pain. Storage and prescription are subject to D.D.A. regulations. *Side effects*: nausea, vomiting, depressed respiration.

(ii) *Non-addictive analgesics*—Act on peripheral nerve endings, relieve joint pain and muscle spasm, e.g. aspirin, paracetamol ('Panadol'), dihydrocodeine ('DF. 118'), pentazocine ('Fortral').

'Ansolysen'—Pentolinium Tartrate—Lowers blood pressure (see Ganglionic Blockade).

Anti-emetics—Drugs to prevent or relieve vomiting, e.g. hyoscine, antihistamines.

Antihistamines—Drugs originally intended for treatment of *allergy** (skin rashes, nasal congestion) but used during and after anaesthesia for *anti-emetic* and *tranquillising* side effects.

'Arfonad'—Trimetaphan—Lowers blood pressure. Short action. May be given by continuous drip ('Arfonad drip'). (see Ganglion blockade).

'Aramine' (Metaraminol)—Raises blood pressure by constricting blood vessels. (See Vasopressors).

'Atarax'—Hydroxyzine—(See Tranquillisers).

Atropine—Active principle of Belladonna ('Deadly Nightshade'.) Depresses vagal activity.

Uses

(*a*) Injected before anaesthesia to dry secretions in mouth and throat, and to prevent slowing of heart during anaesthesia, (*b*) before injection of neostigmin to reverse paralysis due to curare and similar drugs (p. 9). Also dilates pupils and increases pulse rate.

Avomine—Combination of *promethazine* ('Phenergan') and *theoclate* (cerebral stimulant) which antagonises hypnotic side effects of promethazine when used to prevent allergy, nausea, or travel sickness.

Barbiturates—Group of compounds with sleep-inducing (hypnotic) properties but which, when given to those in pain, promote restlessness. Sometimes classified as *rapid* acting, e.g. Quinalbarbitone, Pentobarbitone; *medium* acting, e.g. Butobarbitone; *long* acting, e.g. Phenobarbitone.

Overdose—Unconsciousness with depressed respiration and circulation.

Treatment—Gastric lavage, respiratory stimulants, mechanical ventilation (p. 163).

Bemegride ('Megimide')—Respiratory stimulant for intravenous injection.

'Brietal' (Methohexitone)—Short acting intravenous barbiturate anaesthetic.

Bupivacaine ('Marcain')—Local anaesthetic.

Butobarbitone ('Soneryl')—Barbiturate hypnotic.

Butyrophenones ('Droleptan') = droperidol, ('Serenace') = haloperiodol—Tranquillisers inducing a marked state of indifference. See Neuroleptanalgesia.

Carbromal ('Adalin')—Non-barbiturate hypnotic.

'Carbrital'—Hypnotic containing carbromal and quinalbarbitone.

* *Allergy*: Sensitivity to foreign proteins—dust, pollen, bacterial toxins which cause release of histamine in the tissues.

'Cardiazol' ('Metrazol', 'Leptazol'), Pentamethylene tetrazole—a respiratory stimulant.

Calcium Chloride or Gluconate (5 ml of 10% solution)—'ionised' calcium given i.v. during massive blood transfusion (p. 83).

Chloral Hydrate—Non-barbiturate hypnotic. Unpleasant and nauseating. More palatable preparations are di-chloral phenazone ('Welldorm'), triclofos ('Trichloryl').

Chlordiazepoxide ('Librium')—Tranquilliser.

Chlorhexidine ('Hibitane') — Non-irritant disinfectant. 1% aqueous solution used to disinfect anaesthetic equipment (p. 97).

Chlorpromazine ('Largactil', 'Megaphen', 'Thorazine' (U.S.))—Major tranquilliser with anti-emetic and shock preventing properties. Prolongs action of opiates and anaesthetics.

Cinchocaine ('Nupercaine')—Long acting local anaesthetic, (p. 167).

Cocaine—Addictive local anaesthetic subject to D.D.A. regulations. For *surface application only* (pp. 167, 169).

Codeine (Methyl morphine)—Addictive analgesic derived from opium. Tab. Codeine Co. = aspirin and codeine for pain relief.

'Coramine' (Nikethamide)—Respiratory stimulant.

Cortisone—Preparation of active principle of adrenal cortex for i.m. injection.

Curare (Tubo-curarine chloride, 'Tubarine')—Muscle relaxant. Active principle of South American arrow poison. Now prepared synthetically.

Cyclopropane—Gaseous inhalational anaesthetic stored in RED cylinders (Ch. 4). Inflammable, and with oxygen, explosive.

Decamethonium Iodide ('Syncurine')—Depolarising muscle relaxant (p. 8).

'Demerol' ('Meperidine' (U.S.N.F.))—Synthetic addictive analgesic —see Pethidine.

Dextran ('Dextraven')—Intravenous fluid for treatment of shock (p. 82).

Dextro-Amphetamine ('Dexedrine')—Amphetamine derivative (see Vasopressors).

D.F. 118—Dihydro-codeine non-addictive analgesic.

Diazepam—See 'Valium'.

Digitalis—Cardiac stimulant in treatment of heart failure.

Dimenhydrinate ('Dramamine')—Prevention of nausea and travel sickness (see Antihistamines).

Droperidol ('Droleptan')—Butyrophenone tranquilliser (see Neuroleptanalgesia).

Edrophonium ('Tensilon')—Drug with anticholinesterase action of shorter duration than prostigmin, used to distinguish between muscle weakness due to competitive blockade or depolarisation (p. 8).

'Efcortesol'—Hydrocortisone di-sodium phosphate in solution for i.v. injection (p. 18). Has largely replaced Hydrocortisone di-sodium succinate ('Efcortelan'), a powder requiring solution in water before use.

'Epontol'—Intravenous anaesthetic.

Fentanyl ('Sublimaze')—Synthetic addictive analgesic (see also Neuroleptanalgesia.)

'Fentazine' (Perphenazine)—Anti-emetic (see Antihistamine).

'Flaxedil' (gallamine tri-ethiodide)—Synthetic muscle relaxant of curare type (p. 8).

'Fluothane' (Halothane)—Non-inflammable liquid inhalation anaesthetic (p. 4).

'Fortral' (Pentazocine) Powerful non-addictive analgesic.

Frusemide ('Lasix')—Diuretic.

Ganglionic Blockade—Lowering of blood pressure by drugs which block passage of vasoconstrictor impulses through sympathetic ganglia (ganglion blockers). Used during anaesthesia to lower blood pressure in order to reduce operative haemorrhage by 'controlled hypotension'.

Halothane ('Fluothane')—Non-inflammable liquid anaesthetic (p. 4).

Heparin—Prevents blood clotting. Used for this purpose during arterial surgery. Supplied in multidose bottles containing either *5,000* units or *1,000* units per ml for i.v. injection, hence *careful check of dose is advisable before injection.*

Heroin (diamorphine)—Addictive analgesic related to Morphine.

'Hibitane'—(See Chlorhexidine). Disinfectant.

Hyaluronidase ('Hyalase')—Enzyme which speeds absorption of fluid injected subcutaneously.

Hydrocortisone—Preparation of active principle of cortex of suprarenal gland for i.v. use (p. 18).

Hydrocortisone Sodium Phosphate—'Efcortesol'.

Hydroxyzine ('Atarax', 'Vistaril')—Tranquilliser.

Hyoscine ('Scopolamine')—'Drying' agent with amnesic properties used in pre-operative medication (p. 21).

Hypnotics—Drugs which induce *sleep* but have no pain relieving (analgesic) properties. Two main classes—*Barbiturates* and *Non-barbiturates.*

Inderal (propanolol)—β-adrenergic blocker. Specific action for correction of irregularity of heart beat, e.g. 'extra systoles'.

'Intraval' (thiopentone)—Intravenous anaesthetic.

Isoprenaline ('Isuprel')—Synthetic vasopressor with action resembling adrenaline:

(*a*) *Inhalation* relieves bronchitis, asthma.

(*b*) *Injection* restores circulation during shock by stimulating the heart. Does not cause vasoconstriction.

'Largactil'—See Chlorpromazine.

'Lasix' (Frusemide)—Diuretic.

'Lethidrone' (Nalorphine)—See Morphine antagonists.

Levallorphan ('Lorfan')—See Morphine antagonists.

'Levophed'—See Nor-adrenaline.

'Librium' (Chlordiazepoxide)—Tranquilliser.

Lignocaine ('Xylocaine')—Local anaesthetic (p. 167).

'Lomodex'—Dextraven.

'Lorfan'—See Levallorphan.

'Mandrax'—Non-barbiturate hypnotic containing Methqualone and diphenhydramine.

Mannitol—Intravenous fluid to promote urine flow (p. 82).

'Marcain' (bupivacaine)—Local anaesthetic (p. 167).

'Megimide' (bemegride)—Respiratory stimulant.

'Melsedin'—See Methqualone.

'Meperidine (U.S.N.F.)' (pethidine, demerol)—Synthetic addictive analgesic.

'Mephine' (methenteramine)—Raises blood pressure by constricting blood vessels (see Vasopressors).

Methadone ('Physeptone')—Synthetic addictive analgesic.

'Methedrine' (methylamphetamine)—Raises blood pressure by central stimulation of vasomotor areas in brain (see vasopressors).

Methoxamine ('Vasoxine')—Raises blood pressure by constricting blood vessels (see Vasopressors).

Methqualone ('Melsedin')—Non-barbiturate hypnotic.

Methyl Amphetamine ('Methedrine')—Derivative of amphetamine (see Vasopressors).

Methyl Pentynol ('Oblivon')—Non-barbiturate hypnotic.

Morphine—Addictive analgesic derived from opium.

Morphine Antagonists ('Levallorphan', 'Nalorphine')—Drugs which reverse respiratory depression arising from *addictive analgesics*. Ineffective against respiratory depression from other causes (p. 176).

Nalorphine ('Lethidrone')—See Morphine Antagonists.

Narcotic—Denotes a *central nervous depressant* drug which induces *sleep* (*hypnosis*) and relieves *pain* (*analgesia*). Whilst hypnotics lack pain relieving properties, addictive analgesics, by relieving pain, often induce sleep. Hence (in the U.S.A. particularly) the term is often used to denote any addictive analgesic.

'Nembutal' (pentobarbitone)—Barbiturate hypnotic.

Neostigmin ('Prostigmin')—Anti-cholinesterase for reversal of paralysis from curare (p. 8).

'Neosynephrine' (phenylephrine)—Raises blood pressure by vasoconstriction (see vasopressors).

Nepenthe—Oral preparation of total alkaloids of opium used for pain relief and pre-operative medication of children.

Neuroleptic—Continental term for tranquilliser.

Neuroleptanalgesia—A condition of indifference and insensitivity to pain induced by intravenous injection of a butyrophenone tranquilliser (neuroleptic), droperidol or haloperidol, and a potent analgesic (phenoperidine or fentanyl). May be used during procedures under local analgesia or radiological procedures, or to ensure rapid recovery from general anaesthesia.

Nikethamide ('Coramine')—Respiratory stimulant.

Nitrezepam ('Mogadon')—Non-barbiturate hypnotic.

Nitrous Oxide—Gaseous anaesthetic (p. 3) with analgesic properties.

Nor-adrenaline ('Levophed')—Present in adrenal medulla and released with adrenaline at sympathetic nerve endings. Potent vasoconstrictor. *Nor-adrenaline drip*—4–5 ml nor-adrenaline per litre saline, given at 15–30 drops per minute to raise blood pressure.

Note

(*a*) May induce intense vasoconstriction which can cause gangrene of fingers.

(*b*) Tolerance follows prolonged administration.

(*c*) Circulatory collapse may follow *sudden* withdrawal of nor adrenaline.

Novocaine ('procaine')—Local anaesthetic (p. 167).

'Nupercaine' (cinchocaine)—Long acting local anaesthetic (p. 167).

'Oblivon' (methyl pentynol)—Non-barbiturate hypnotic.

'Omnopon'—Addictive analgesic. See Papaveretum, B.P.

'Operidine'—See phenoperidine.

'Panadol'—See paracetamol.

Papaveretum B.P. ('Omnopon', 'Pantopon')—Addictive analgesic containing 50% Morphine, 50% Opium alkaloids.

Papaverine—Opium alkaloid which relaxes smooth (involuntary) muscles, following direct application (1 in 40). Used to *overcome spasm of arteries* arising from injury, irritation (e.g. injection of thiopentone), or before inserting cannulae.

Paracetamol ('Panadol')—Non-addictive analgesic.

Paraldehyde—Non-barbiturate hypnotic with unpleasant smell. Effective by rectal route and by i.m. injection.

Pentobarbitone ('Nembutal')—Rapid acting barbiturate hypnotic.

Pentolinium ('Ansolysen')—Lowers blood pressure (see Ganglionic Blockade).

'Pentothal' ('Intraval', thiopentone)—Intravenous barbiturate anaesthetic (p. 3).

Pentazocine—See 'Fortral'.

Perphenazine ('Fentazin')—Prevents nausea and vomiting (see Phenothiazines).

Pethidine ('Demerol', Meperidine U.S.N.F.)—Synthetic addictive analgesic.

'Pethilorfan'—Mixture of Pethidine and Levallorphan (p. 176).

'Phenergan' (promethazine)—Phenothiazine derivative with pronounced anti-histamine property.

Phenobarbitone—Long acting barbiturate hypnotic. Calming action in small dose.

Phenoperidine ('Operidine')—Potent addictive analgesic, see Neuroleptanalgesia.

Phenothiazine Derivatives—Group of drugs which combine tranquillising actions with several other apparently unrelated properties, but all of which arise from depression of the brain stem reticular formation. These include:

(*a*) Intensification of action of hypnotics, analgesics, anaesthetics.
(*b*) Anti-emetic action.
(*c*) Anti-tussive (cough preventing) action.
(*d*) Reduction of blood pressure.
(*e*) Shock prevention.
(*f*) Reduction of muscle tone.

Uses:

(i) To prevent nausea and vomiting.
(ii) Combined with analgesics or hypnotics in pre- and post-operative medication (p. 21).
(iii) To overcome the vasoconstrictor manifestations of shock (p. 117).
(iv) To prevent shivering during induction of hypothermia (p. 164).

Phenylephrine—See 'Neosynephrine'.

'Physeptone' (methadone)—Synthetic addictive analgesic.

'Pitocin'—Oxytocic principle of Posterior Pituitary. Smooth muscle stimulant. 'Pitocin drip' given to overcome delay in childbirth. Incompatible with Cyclopropane.

'Priscol' (tolazoline)—Vasodilator, for 'cold hands and feet'.
Procaine—See 'Novocaine'.
Promazine ('Sparine')—Tranquilliser (see phenothiazines).
Promethazine ('Phenergan')—See phenothiazines and 'Phenergan'.
Propanidid—See 'Epontol'.
Propanolol—See 'Inderal'.
'Prostigmin'—See Neostigmine.
Quinalbarbitone ('Seconal')—Quick acting barbiturate hypnotic.
Respiratory stimulants—Drugs to stimulate depressed respiration, e.g. 'Nikethamide', aminophylline, 'Cardiazol', bemegride.
'Rheomacrodex'—Dextran (p. 82).
'Scoline' (succinyl choline, suxamethonium)—Depolarising muscle relaxant (p. 8).
'Scopolamine'—See Hyoscine.
'Seconal' (Quinalbarbitone)—Rapid acting barbiturate hypnotic.
Sedative—Drugs which allay activity and excitement by depression of the central nervous system. A general term, which does not differentiate between *analgesic*, *hypnotic*, and *tranquillising* actions.
'Soneryl' (Butobarbitone)—Medium acting barbiturate hypnotic.
'Sparine' (Promazine)—Tranquilliser (see phenothiazines).
Steroids—Secretions of adrenal cortex (p. 18).
'Sublimaze' (Fentanyl)—Powerful addictive analgesic (see 'Neuroleptanalgesia').
Succinyl Choline—See 'Scoline'.
Suxamethonium—See 'Scoline'.
'Syncurine'—Decamethonium Iodide. Depolarising muscle relaxant (p. 8).
Tacrine ('T.H.A.', tetra-amino-acrine, 'Romotal')—Weak anticholinesterase drug like neostigmine. Prolongs action of scoline and other depolarising relaxants.
'Tensilon'—See edrophonium.
'Thalamol'—Mixture of fentanyl and droperidol (see Neuroleptanalgesia).
Thiopentone ('Pentothal', 'Intraval')—Intravenous anaesthetics.
Toxiferine ('Alloferin')—Competitive muscle relaxant.
Tranquillisers—Drugs which allay anxiety and induce a tranquil frame of mind without sleepiness or clouding of consciousness ('day-time sedatives').
Tribromethanol (Bromethol, 'Avertin')—Strong hypnotic drug formerly given by rectal route to induce unconsciousness before anaesthesia. Sometimes given to control convulsions, due to toxaemia of pregnancy.
Tricloryl ('Triclofos')—Palatable preparation of *chloral*.
Trimeprazine—See 'Vallergan'.

Trimetaphan—See 'Arfonad'.

Trichlorethylene ('Trilene')—Liquid inhalational anaesthetic with strong analgesic action in subanaesthetic doses (p. 178).

'Tubarine' (Tubocurarine chloride)—Muscle relaxant, see Curare.

'Valium' (diazepam)—Hypnotic with anti-convulsive properties.

'Vallergan' (trimeprazine)—Phenothiazine derivative resembling promethazine ('Phenergan') prepared in syrup form ('Vallergan Elixir') as palatable pre-operative medication for children.

'Vandid' (Vanillic acid di-ethylamide)—Intravenous respiratory stimulant. Available in drop form to stimulate respiration in the new-born.

Vasopressors—Drugs administered to raise systolic blood pressure. All (*except Ephedrine*) are chemically related to Adrenaline. They produce their effects by:

(*a*) Stimulation of vasomotor centres in the brain (central action).
(*b*) Stimulation of the heart muscle.
(*c*) Constriction of peripheral blood vessels (vasoconstrictor action).

Vasopressors which have a strong central action (e.g. *amphetamines*) in addition increase wakefulness, lessen sense of fatigue, reduce appetite and cause insomnia.

Use of vasopressors:

(i) To counteract fall in blood pressure due to spinal or epidural anaesthesia.
(ii) To reverse the hypotensive action of adrenolytic drugs.
(iii) In treatment of shock (p. 117) and of barbiturate poisoning.

'Vasoxine' (methoxamine)—Vasopressor effective mainly through vasoconstriction.

'Vinesthene' (di-vinyl ether)—Inhalational anaesthetic for short procedures.

'Vistaril' ('Atarax')—See hydroxyzine.

'Welldorm' (di-chloral phenazone)—Non-barbiturate hypnotic.

Xylocaine—See lignocaine.

INDEX

Further references to drugs will be found in Chapter 22 (page 182).

Acetyl choline, in neuromuscular transmission, 6–8
Adrenaline
in anaphylactic shock, 147
in cardiac arrest, 155
in local anaesthesia, 170
in ventricular fibrillation, 147
Adverse reaction to anaesthetics, drugs and, 17
Airway caps, 54
Airway props, 55
Airways, 53
disinfection of, 97
Ambu Hesse non-return valve, 71
Ambu self-inflating bag, 150, 155
Amethocaine, 167, 168, 183
Analgesia in midwifery, 176–178
Anaphylactic shock, 147
Anti-emetics, 28, 184
'Atarax', 21, 184
Atropine, 21, 23, 184
Ayre's 'T' piece, 65, 70–72

Barbiturates, 21, 184
dosage for children, 23
in childbirth, 176
poisoning treatment of, 163
Beaver Jointed Tracheostomy Connector, 139
Blood loss, measurement of, 88
Blood pressure
after coronary thrombosis, 163
after head injuries, 164
during recovery, 109, 111–112
during shock, 119
following steroids, 117
in anaphylactic shock, 147
in barbiturate poisoning, 164
in epidural and spinal anaesthesia, 174
measurement of, 85
vasodilators and, 117
vasopressors and, 117
Blood transfusion
checking of blood, 83–84
equipment for, 79–81
hazards of massive transfusion, 83
in shock and haemorrhage, 116
storage of blood, 83
Blood volume, measurement of, 88
Bosun Warning Device, 37–41
Boyle's apparatus, 30–31, 42
Brain
action of anaesthetics on, 2
consciousness and, 11
'Brietal' (see methohexital)
British Standard fittings, 42, 43, 49
Bronchoscopes, 68–69
Brook airway, 149–152, 154
Bupivacaine, 167, 168, 184
Butyrophenones, 21, 184
in local analgesia, 21
in neuroleptanalgesia, 188

Carbon dioxide
absorption of, 46–49
analysis of, 87
colour of cylinders, 30
sterilisation of absorbers, 98
use during anaesthesia, 31
Carbon monoxide poisoning, 131
treatment by hyperbaric oxygen, 131
Cardiac arrest
causes, 146
defibrillator for, 154–155
definition, 146
diagnosis, 147-148
drugs for, 155
electrocardiograph for, 154–155
equipment for treatment, 154–155
external cardiac massage, 151–152
infusion sodium bicarbonate, 154–155
insufflation with Brook airway, 149-152, 154
mouth to mouth respiration, 148
objects of treatment, 153

Cardiac arrest (*contd.*)
organisation for emergency treatment, 153
pacemaker in, 147–155
self-inflating bags, 150–152
Cardiac arrest box, 154
Cardiff attachment, 45
Cardiff inflating bellows, 150, 155
Cardioscope, 87
Caudal needles, 171–172
Central Midwives Board, 178–179
Childbirth, analgesia and anaesthesia for,
apparatus for self-administration, 177-178
checking apparatus, 178
choice of face mask, 178
legal requirements, 179
technique of administration, 179
drugs for analgesia, 176
general anaesthesia, hazards of, 180
indications for, 180
precautionary measures, 180–181
preparation of apparatus, 180
inhalational anaesthesia, 176
local anaesthesia
pudendal block, 181
regional blocks, 181
psycho-physical preparation, 175
Children and infants, 69–73
Chlordiazepoxide, 21, 185
Chloroform, 176
Chlorpromazine, 21, 185
in hypepyrexia, 164
in shock prevention, 117
in shock treatment, 117
route of injection, 22
Cholinesterase, in neuromuscular transmission, 6–8
Cinchocaine, 167, 168, 185
Clausen's Harness, 45
Cocaine, 68, 167, 168, 169, 185
Codeine compound, 28, 185
Connell's Harness, 45
Consent forms, 25
Corney visual suction end, 52
disinfection of, 97
Curare, 7–8
Cut-down sets, 78
Cyclopropane cylinders, 30–31
explosions with, 90

Day patients, 26–28
Decamethonium, 8
Defibrillator in cardiac arrest, 154–155
Dehydration, 19
Diabetes, 16, 17
Diazepam, 21, 174
Diazepoxide, 21
Disposable intravenous cannulae, 76–78

East Freeman non-return valve, 71
Electrocardiograph
after cardiac surgery, 163
for pre-operative assessment, 14
in cardiac arrest, 154–155
in coronary thrombosis, 14, 163
principles of, 87
'Emotril', the, 178
Endotracheal, anaesthesia
adaptor, mounts, 65–66
adaptor tubes, 44, 65–66
definition, 10, 59
equipment for, 59
local anaesthetic sprays, 68, 93, 95, 154
Endotracheal connections, 67–68, 93
Endotracheal tubes, 11, 61–65, 93, 97
Epidural anaesthesia, 171–174
during childbirth, 181
'Epontol', 3, 190
Ether, 4
inflammability, 90
'Eulissin', 8
'Entonox' the, 177
Expiratory valve, 44

Face masks, 44
cleaning and disinfection, 97
Fire and explosions, 90–91
'Flaxedil', 8, 186
'Fluotec', 36
'Fluothane', 4, 6, 18, 36 (see halothane)
Frenchay Hospital suction end, 52
disinfection of, 97

Gallamine, 8, 186
Gas cylinders, 30–35
Gaseous anaesthetics, 3
General anaesthesia
definition, 1
depression of reflex activity, 11
during childbirth, 180, 181
estimation of depth, 11
endotracheal intubation during, 95
for children, 69
for infants, 69

General anaesthesia (*contd.*)
induction of, 94
inhalational, 3–5
intravenous, 3
intravenous induction, 94
maintenance, 5
preparations for, 92
protection of patient during, 99
recovery from, 12, 109–111
types, 2–3
Goldman Inhaler, 36
Gordh Needle, 75

Halothane, 4, 6, 18, 186
vaporisers for, 36
Head injuries, 164
'Hippocratic facies', 19
Holmes, Oliver Wendell, 1
Howard Jones spinal needle, 171, 172
Hydroxyzine, 21, 186
Hyoscine, 21, 186
for children, 23, 2
Hypnotics, 21, 186
Hypotensive drugs,

'Inderal', 163, 186
Indicator discs, 32
Infants (see children)
Intensive Care Unit
administration, 158
advantages, 156
arrangement of, 157
disadvantages, 156
head injury charts, 164
medical supervision, 158
nursing care
general nursing care, 159
turning patient, 158
purposes, 156
special procedures, 159
after cardiac surgery, 162
barbituate poisoning, 163, 164
central venous pressure, 160
coronary thrombosis, 163
drug treatment, 163
fluid balance charts, 159, 160
head injuries, 164
treatment of hyperpyrexia in, 164–165
Intermittent flow machines, 41
'Intraval', 3, 187
Intravenous anaesthesia
common agents, 3
equipment for, 74
induction of, 94
needles for, 75–76
Intravenous infusions, 79, 93
disposable cannulae for, 76–78
equipment for, 79–81
fluids for, 81–84, 155
blood, 83
cut-down sets for, 78, 155
dextran solutions, 82
plasma, 83
solutions of salts and sugars, 81–82
urea, 84
'Intraval' (see thiopentone)

'Ketalar', 3, 187

Labat syringe, 170
'Largactil', 21, 187
route of injection, 22
Laryngoscopes, 59–61, 93
Lee extradural needle, 171, 172
Levallorphan, 176, 187
'Librium', 21, 187
Lignocaine, 167, 187
Liquid anaesthetics, 4
Local anaesthesia
care during local anaesthesia, 173–174
complications of, 174
definition, 1, 166
drugs used, 167, 168
equipment for, 170
in childbirth, 181
local anaesthetic sprays, 68
methods, 168
position for epidural or spinal blocks, 173
use of adrenaline, 170, 174
Local anaesthetics, 167, 168 (see local anaesthesia)
Lorfan (see levallorphan)

Mackintosh laryngoscope, 59
Mackintosh spray, 68
Magill breathing attachment, 42, 43
Magill laryngoscope, 59
Magill, Sir Ivan, 10, 42
Magill's tubes, 10, 61
endotracheal connections, 67
endotracheal introducing forceps, 65–66, 93
flexometallic tube, 64
introducer, 172–173
'Marcain', 167, 168, 187
Marrett's anaesthetic apparatus, 39, 41
'M.C. oxygen mask', 128

'Medatron' blood loss meter, 88
Methohexital, 3
Methoxyfluorane, 5
'M.I.E.' Temperature compensated vaporiser, 36
Minnitt, R. J., 177
Minnitt's apparatus, 177
Mitchell Needle, 75
Monitoring equipment, 85, 90
  use in intensive care, 162–163
Monoamine oxidase inhibitors, 17–18
Morphine, 21, 187
  in coronary thrombosis, 163
Mouth gags, 57, 58
  disinfection of, 97
Mouth props, 55, 56
Mouth wedge, 55, 57
  disinfection of, 97
'Multicaine', spray, 68
Muscle relaxants, 5–8

National Physical Laboratory, 178
Neostigmin, 8, 188
  anticholinesterase action, 8, 9
  atropine and, 9
Neuromuscular transmission, 6–7
Nitrous oxide
  apparatus for use in childbirth, 177
  cylinders, 30, 32
  pressure gauges, 34, 35
Nosworthy endotracheal connection, 67
Novocaine, 167, 168, 188
'Nupercaine', 167, 168, 188

Odom's indicator, 172, 173
Omnopon, 21, 188
  for children, 23–24
  in coronary thrombosis, 163
Operating suite, communications with, 26, 107
Opiates, 21, 176, 183
Oxygen
  combustion from, 90
  cylinders, 30
  hyperbaric
    care of patients, 133
    complications, 133
    emergency supply, 37
    indications for, 131–133
    methods of administration, 132–133
    theory of, 131
  therapy
    carbon dioxide retention in, 127–130
    equipment, 127–129
    flow rates for, 131
    indications for, 127

Pacemakers, artificial, 147, 155
'Pamergan', 21
'Panadol', 28, 183, 189
Pancuronium, 8
Papaveretum, 21, 188
  for children, 23–24
  in coronary thrombosis, 163
Paracetamol, 28, 183, 189
Paraldehyde, 24, 189
'Pavulon' (see pancuronium)
'Penthrane' (see methoxyfluorane)
'Pentothal', 3, 189
  rectal administration, 24
Pethilorfan, 176, 189
Pethine, 21, 176, 189
  during local anaesthesia, 123
  in coronary thrombosis, 163
'Phenergan' (see promethazine)
Phenothiazines, 21, 189
Physiotherapy
  during respiratory failure, 144
  pre-operative, 15
  post-operative, 15
Pin-index system, 33–34
Position of patient on operating table, 99–102
Pre-anaesthetic medication, 20 (see premedication)
Premedication, 21–25
Pre-operative assessment (see also preparation of patient)
  anaemia and, 16
  for elective surgery, 13
  for emergency surgery, 18–19
  metabolic conditions, 16
  of cardiovascular system, 13–14
  of respiratory system, 15
  purpose of, 13
  significance of drug treatment in, 17
Preparation of patient, 20
  anaemia, 16
  breathing exercises, 15
  cardiovascular system, 13
  consent forms, 25
  day of operation, 24
  dentures and valuables, 25
  empty stomach, 24
  for emergency surgery, 18–19
  in dehydration, 19
  in shock, 19

Preparation of patient (*contd.*)
metabolic conditions, 16, 17
of children, 22
postural drainage, 15
pre-operative injection, 21
respiratory function tests, 16
respiratory system, 15
smoking, 15–16
Pressure indicator gauges, 33, 34
Procaine, 167, 168, 190
Promazine (see 'Sparine')
Promethazine, 21, 190
dose for children, 23
in childbirth, 176
in local anaesthesia, 174
route of injection, 22
Propanidid, 3, 190
Propanolol, 163, 190
'Prostigmin' (see neostigmin)
Pseudocholinesterase, 9
Psycho-physical preparation, 175
Psychoprophylaxis, 175
Pulsometers, 86

Recovery,
complications of, 113–117
nursing procedure in, 107–112
Recovery room, 105–107
Rectal premedication, 24
Reducing valves, 33
Reid, Grantley Dick, 175
Rendell-Baker infant's mask, 72–73
Respiration, 118–123
Respiratory failure, 124–128
treatment of, 127–129
treatment with ventilators, 134–137
Respiratory function tests, 16
Rotameters, 35
Rowbotham, Sidney, 10
Rowbotham's endotracheal connection, 67
Ruben non-return valve, 70
Ryle's (naso-gastric) tube, 109

Schimmelbusch mask, 69
'Scoline' (see suxamethonium)
Scopolamine, 21, 190
for children, 23–24
Shock, 19, 115–117
Simpson, James Young, 176
Sise introducer, 172–173
Soda lime, 50–51
'Sparine', 21, 190
in childbirth, 176
in coronary thrombosis, 153
in hyperpyrexia, 164
route of injection, 22
Spinal anaesthesia, 171–174, 181
Spirometer the, 16
Sterilisation of equipment, 96–97
Steroids, 17–18
Subdural anaesthesia, 171 (see spinal anaesthesia)
Suction, 51–53
Suxamethonium, 7–8, 10
'Syncurine' (see decamethonium)

'Tecota', 178
Thiopentone, 3, 190
rectal administration, 24
Tongue forceps, 56–57
'Toxiferine', 8, 190
Tracheostomy, 138–144
Tranquillisers, 20–21, 190
for children, 23
in childbirth, 176
in coronary thrombosis, 163
in epidural anaesthesia, 174
in hyperbaric oxygen therapy, 133
in premedication, 21
in treatment with ventilators, 136
Trichlorethylene, 4, 190
in midwifery, 178, 177
vaporisers for, 178
'Trilene' (see trichlorethylene)
Trimeprazine, 23, 190
'Tubarine' (see tubocurarine)
Tuohy needle, 171–172

'Valium', 21, 191, 174
'Vallergan', 23, 190
Vaporisers, 4, 36, 178
Vaso-vagal syndrome, 174
Venous pressure, 85–86, 160–162
Ventilators, 134–137 (see also respiratory failure)
use with tracheostomy, 142–143
'Ventimask', 129
Vitalograph, the, 16
'Volemetron', 88

Walton five anaesthetic apparatus, 40
Waters, Ralph, 46
Waters' canister, 46, 47
sterilisation of, 98
Wright respirometer, 88–89

Xylocaine, 167, 168, 191

Yankauer suction end, 52, 97